Commission of the European Communities

RADIATION PROTECTION RESEARCH
AND TRAINING PROGRAMME

THYROID CANCER IN CHILDREN LIVING NEAR CHERNOBYL

Expert panel report on the consequences of the Chernobyl accident

Edited by

D. Williams,[1] A. Pinchera,[2] A. Karaoglou,[3] K. H. Chadwick[3]

[1] University of Cambridge
Department of Histopathology
Addenbrooke's Hospital
Hills Road
Cambridge CB2 2QQ
United Kingdom

[2] Istituto di Endocrinologia
Universita degli Studi di Pisa
Viale del Tirreno, 64
I-56018 Tirrenia-Pisa

[3] Directorate-General XII/F-6
Science, Research and Development
ARTS-LUX
200, rue de la Loi
B-1049 Brussels

Directorate-General
Science, Research and Development

1993

EUR 15248 EN

Published by the
COMMISSION OF THE EUROPEAN COMMUNITIES
Directorate-General XIII
Telecommunications, Information Market and Exploitation of Research

L-2920 Luxembourg

Cataloguing data can be found at the end of this publication

Luxembourg: Office for Official Publications of the European Communities, 1993

ISBN 92-826-5515-6

Printed in France

Contents

		Page
Preface		v
1.	Consensus Opinion	1
2.	Introduction	3
3.	Motivation	4
4.	Context	7
5.	The Thyroid, Iodine Isotopes and Cancer	13
	5.1 Physiology of thyroid; role of iodine	13
	5.2 Iodine isotopes released in a nuclear accident	14
	5.3 Radiation-induced thyroid cancer	18
6.	The reactor accident in Chernobyl and subsequent thyroid doses	22
7.	Thyroid cancer in children after the Chernobyl accident	32
	7.1 Present evidence related to Chernobyl	32
	7.2 Pathology Confirmation	39
8.	Prevention, Diagnosis and Management of disease	46
9.	Projection of possible future developments	53
10.	Current International actions	60
	10.1 WHO	61
	10.2 WHO Europe	62
	10.3 USA	64
	10.4 Japan	66
	10.5 Germany	69
	10.6 The Netherlands	71
	10.7 Switzerland	73
	10.8 France	75

11. **Recommendations - Actions** 76

    11.A.   Technical Assistance 76

        A.1. Aims 76

        A.2. Realisation 77

        A.3. Diagnosis of thyroid cancer in children 78

        A.4. Treatment of thyroid cancer in children 79

        A.5. Follow-up of thyroid cancer in children 80

        A.6. Iodine deficiency 80

    11.B.   Research cooperation in the development of skills

                       between the CIS and the CEC 82

        B.1. Development of protocols for treatment 82

        B.2. The molecular, cellular and biological characterisation

                of childhood thyroid tumours 83

    11.C.   Coordination of the various Chernobyl related studies . . . 90

12. **Conclusions** 91

References 95

Acknowledgements 100

Annex : Glossary 101

Preface

In January 1992, the Radiation Protection Research Action formed a Panel of Thyroid Experts in order to evaluate the current situation concerning reported increased rates of thyroid cancer in children living in the neighbourhood of Chernobyl at the time of the nuclear reactor accident which occurred on April 26, 1986. *This panel consisted of the following individuals:*

Prof. Sir Dillwyn Williams	*Cambridge University, UK*
Prof. A. Pinchera	*Pisa University, Italy*
Prof. B. Egloff	*Kantonsspital Winterthur, Switzerland*
Prof. C. Reiners	*Essen University, Germany*
Dr. P. Fragu	*INSERM, France*
Dr. K. Baverstock	*WHO Europe, Rome Division, Italy*

The Panel Members together with the *CEC Officials K.H. Chadwick and A. Karaoglou of the Radiation Protection Research Action of the Directorate General XII "Science, Research and Development",* visited Minsk in October 1992. In order to facilitate International collaboration, invitations were issued to Japanese and American authorities to send observers to the Panel meeting in Minsk. *Prof. S. Nagataki, Nagasaki University, from Japan, and Dr. B.W. Wachholz, NCI, Washington, together with Dr. J. Robbins, NIH, Bethesda, and Dr. D.V. Becker, Cornell Medical Centre, New York, from the USA* consequently participated as observers representing their respective countries. In addition *Professor Th. Abelin, Berne University, Switzerland, and Dr. J. Notenboom, ITRI-TNO, The Netherlands,* also joined the Panel as observers.

Thanks to the helpful cooperation of the Ministry of Health of Belarus the Panel and Observers were able to examine patients, talk with Belarus scientists and participate in a Symposium on Chernobyl and Thyroid Cancer.

This report documents the findings of the Panel with respect to the occurrence of childhood thyroid cancer in Belarus after the Chernobyl reactor accident as of November 1992 and makes strong recommendations for urgent Technical and Humanitarian Assistance and Research Cooperation.

The Radiation Protection Research Action of the Energy Programme of the Directorate General for Science, Research and Development of the Commission of the European Communities and the Members of the Thyroid Expert Panel wish to acknowledge the tremendous help of all the Belarus scientists whose willing cooperation made this report possible, and more especially:

His Excellency, Dr. V. S. Kazakov, Minister of Health of Belarus; Dr. N.A. Krysenko, Deputy Minister of Health; Prof. E.P. Demidchik; Prof. L.N. Astakhova; Prof. E. Cherstvoy; Dr. A.W. Furmanchuk; Dr. V.A. Matyuchin; Dr. J.I. Averkin, all their collaborators and Mrs. N.M. Ievleva.

The open collaboration and the warm hospitality offered to the Panel Members, CEC Officials and International Observers on their mission to Belarus were very appreciated.

Thanks are also due to all the International Observers who gave so freely of their time to participate in the mission and have contributed so readily to the realisation of this document.

<table>
<tr><td>H. Allgeier</td><td>J. Sinnaeve</td></tr>
<tr><td>Director</td><td>Head of Unit</td></tr>
<tr><td>Energy Programme</td><td>Radiation Protection</td></tr>
</table>

1. Consensus opinion

The Panel accepts that in the years since the Chernobyl accident, there has been a substantial increase in the incidence of thyroid carcinoma in children in Southern Belarus. The pathological diagnosis of the great majority of cases has been independently confirmed. Recently, a considerable increase in childhood thyroid cancer has also been reported in Northern Ukraine.

The pathological evidence shows that the tumours are virtually all papillary carcinomas and are relatively aggressive, with the majority of cases showing direct invasion of extra-thyroid tissues, and lymph node spread. The majority of the children examined (26 children) personally by Panel members had presented by non-screening routes. This observation leads the Panel to conclude that greater awareness and ascertainment are unlikely to account for much of the increase in cancer incidence.

Evidence to date suggests that the most likely cause of this increase in childhood thyroid cancer is the Chernobyl nuclear reactor accident on April 26, 1986. This evidence includes the geographical distribution and the temporal occurrence of the cancer cases.

The Chernobyl reactor accident was unprecedented in scale and in the size of the population exposed. Very large amounts of radioactivity including isotopes of iodine were released from the reactor. Previous data indicate that increased thyroid carcinoma incidence has followed exposure to direct radiation or to radioactive fallout from the detonation of nuclear weapons. Children have been shown to be more susceptible than adults to the carcinogenic effect of radiation to the thyroid. The radiation dose to the thyroid from isotopes of iodine would be increased in areas of iodine deficiency, such as are found in the regions surrounding Chernobyl. The Panel considers that radioactive isotopes of iodine released from the damaged reactor are the most likely cause of the post-Chernobyl increase in childhood thyroid cancer found in Belarus and the Ukraine.

The Panel recognises that it is not possible to predict the future extent of the incidence of thyroid cancer and therefore considers that long-term monitoring of the exposed population is necessary. The Panel recommends that urgent action be taken at the public health level to provide assistance for diagnosis and treatment of thyroid cancer and at the scientific level, to increase the understanding of the aetiology of thyroid cancers.

Panel Members	**International Observers**
Prof. Sir Dillwyn Williams	*Dr. D. Becker*
Prof. A. Pinchera	*Dr. J. Robbins*
Prof. B. Egloff	*Dr. B. Wachholz*
Prof. C. Reiners	*Prof. S. Nagataki*
Dr. P. Fragu	*Prof. Th. Abelin*
Dr. K. Baverstock	*Dr. J. Notenboom*

CEC Officials

Dr. K.H. Chadwick

Dr. A. Karaoglou

2. Introduction

The Panel first met at GSF-Forschungszentrum für Umwelt und Gesundheit, Münich, on January 15, 1992, at the invitation of *Professor A. Kellerer*, to discuss reports of an excess of childhood thyroid cancer in the Minsk region of Belarus. There were 15 participants including two scientists from Minsk, Belarus, *Professor L.N. Astakhova* and *Dr. V. Drost*, and Commission officials. The experts were initially sceptical of the reported increase of childhood thyroid cancer, but following a presentation by *Professor L. N. Astakhova*, it became clear that there was substance to the claims and that it was necessary to confirm the validity of the data by an independent international body of scientists. It was recommended that EC experts should reassess the pathology of the cases, review case notes, and receive the most appropriate material for histological examination. Most of the members of the Panel met together with *Dr. A. W. Furmanchuk* from Minsk, and Commission officials in Dublin on June 22 - 23, 1992, and were convinced, after viewing a series of 35 mm slides made by *Professor B. Egloff* from microscopic examination of thyroid tissue samples from Belarus, of the validity of the pathological diagnosis. The Panel was also presented with data on the age distribution of the first 100 cases at the time of the accident and at the time of diagnosis. It was decided that the CEC Panel of Experts would meet in Minsk, together with the International Observers on October 25-31, 1992. The aim of this mission was to examine the data and the available patients, and to make a thorough assessment of the newer cases. In Minsk the Panel defined future needs and actions which will aid these children, drafted recommendations and arrived at a consensus opinion. This Consensus Opinion forms the introductory statement to this report. On December 21 - 22, 1992, the Panel met in Brussels to finalize the report. This report deals essentially with the occurrence of childhood thyroid cancer in Belarus, but also represents the consensus of the Panel on the current situation relating to post Chernobyl thyroid cancer in children in the three republics.

3. Motivation

The Chernobyl reactor accident occurred on April 26 1986 and resulted in widespread radioactive contamination over large areas of Belarus, Russia, Ukraine and, to a lesser extent, the Baltic countries and the rest of Europe. There was concern throughout the population of the European Community because of the potential radiological consequences. The Commission's Radiation Protection Research Action responded immediately by proposing a revision of the Radiation Protection Programme 1985-1989 (COM(87)332 Final) with the specific aim of launching 10 coordinated multinational projects for assessing and mitigating the short-term consequences within the Community. The revision of the Radiation Protection Programme was approved by the Council on December 21, 1987, with a budget of 10 mio ECU (OJ No. L 16/44 of 21.01.88). The studies of the 10 specific lines of research yielded a comprehensive overview of the short-term consequences in the Community and were the first step towards the evaluation of the medium-term consequences. The results from these ten research investigations have been published as a series of EUR Reports and an overview is presented in the EUR Report published in 1990 (EUR 13199).

In 1991, the Communication of the Commission to the Council (SEC(91)220 DEF, 12.02.91) outlined, as part of the continued concern with the consequences of the

Chernobyl accident, the background for a collaboration between the Commission's Research Action and the "Chernobyl Centre for International Research" (CHECIR). This centre was created in the frame of an agreement for international collaboration between the All-Union Ministry for Atomic Power and Industry and the International Atomic Energy Agency. In the frame of the ""Activités complémentaires de préparation, d'accompagnement et de suivi - Collaboration with the former Soviet Union in Radiation Protection" (APAS-COSU) programme, a preparatory phase of 7 projects, dealing with radioecology and nuclear emergency management, was launched. Following the dissolution of the Soviet Union in 1991 the collaboration continued with the Ministries responsible for the mitigation of the consequences of the accident in the three republics Belarus, Russia and the Ukraine.

In 1992, an "Agreement for International Collaboration on the Consequences of the Chernobyl Accident" between the Commission and the representatives of the ministeries of the republics of Belarus, Russia and Ukraine was signed on June 23 by *Vice-President Pandolfi*, providing a formal basis for this cooperation. Following a call for proposals, the 7 projects were extended, and at present 7 multinational teams (with the participation of 45 European research groups) collaborate with multi-state teams from the three republics. Also in 1992, 3 additional projects dealing with the medium-term health consequences of the accident were launched. These concern: "Epidemiology and dose reconstruction"; "Biological dosimetry including cytogenetics"; and "Treatment of accident victims". Further studies will have to be implemented to finalize the medium-term assessments and prepare the evaluation of the long-term consequences. These can only be realized through substantial collaboration with the three republics.

The most important long-term health hazard from radiation exposure is the induction of malignancy and studies of the Atom Bomb survivors in Japan have revealed that the incidence of leukaemia starts to increase some five years after exposure. Consequently, health hazards from the Chernobyl accident are now anticipated and health consequences of the accident are now becoming evident. The major medium-term effects of concern are radiation-induced thyroid cancer and leukaemia. Thyroid cancer has already been observed in children who were evacuated from, or are still living in, areas where significant deposition of radioactivity occurred. Leukaemia is anticipated in the period of 5 to 15 years following the accident especially in those who helped to deal with the reactor fire and the immediate clean-up operations, the so called "liquidators", and in specific population groups. The very long-term health consequences are expected to be the radiation-induced solid cancers which have been found to increase some 20 years after exposure in the Atom Bomb survivors. Their eventual registration for future epidemiological studies requires the urgent establishment of a medical infrastructure and follow-up.

This report deals with the present situation concerning thyroid cancer in children living in the three republics in the regions around Chernobyl with emphasis on the children living in Belarus. It has been written to document the situation at the end of 1992 as assessed by European experts but also to increase scientific and public awareness of the health problem, to initiate action at the public health and scientific level, and is addressed to those with an interest in Radiological Protection and Nuclear Emergency Management. It is also addressed to those responsible for Technical Assistance and Humanitarian Aid in the three republics Belarus, Russia and The Ukraine.

4. Context

Nuclear power generates a considerable proportion of the total energy consumed in the world, especially in the industrialised countries. There are at present almost 400 reactors in the world devoted to civil nuclear power. Almost one third of these are concentrated in the European Community which has a total number greater than the USA and more than twice as many as the Ex-Soviet Union countries. Nuclear power has always been advocated as a clean and safe means of energy production and power reactors have always been designed to be fail-safe such that a review of the engineering safety features of reactors in 1976 concluded that the chance of a serious reactor accident was infinitesimally small. This study did not adequately take into account the problems which can arise in the interaction of human activity and complex engineering systems. The serious reactor accident at Three Mile Island, USA in 1979, while not leading to the off-site release of large amounts of radioactivity, did reveal that the presence of engineering safety features could not exclude completely the possibility of a serious reactor accident. The Chernobyl nuclear power plant accident, the worst of its kind, has re-emphasized the problems that can arise in the event of a possible future accident and has increased concern about the safety of reactors designed in the ex-Soviet Union which do not carry the same level of engineered safety features as those designed and constructed in the West. More specifically the reactors in the Ex-Soviet Union do not have a secondary containment vessel around the core which can help to reduce the amount of radioactivity released to the environment in the case of an accident.

The Chernobyl reactor accident released enormous amounts of radioactive contamination into the atmosphere and caused a widespread contamination over virtually the whole of Europe. Almost all countries of the European community, with the exception of Spain and Portugal, were exposed to the plume of radioactivity. The most highly contaminated regions of the Community were Northern Italy, Southern Germany, and Greece, but even here the highest total body doses to the population (largely from Caesium) were only of the same order as that which is accrued from natural background radiation over a year.

While the risk of an event such as the Chernobyl accident has been widely regarded as sufficiently small, especially after the Three Mile Island accident, some studies on the possible consequences of such a happening have been performed (Evans et al., 1985). In particular, it was widely recognized that, in the case of an accident the more volatile radioactive fission products, such as the isotopes of Caesium and Iodine, would be released as a vapour from the hot reactor fuel. Iodine was seen to pose a specific hazard because it is taken up by the body and concentrated in the thyroid gland. Thus, in the immediate aftermath of a reactor accident which releases the volatile fission products to the atmosphere the thyroid, because of its avidity for iodine, is greatly at risk (Dumont et al., 1980).

The thyroid is a critical organ in the initial phase of radioactive contamination after a reactor accident.

The most important radioactive isotopes of Iodine formed as fission products are short-lived and the radioactivity decays rapidly; for instance, Iodine-131 has a radioactive half life of 8 days so that in about three months the Iodine-131 radioactivity will decrease by a thousand fold. The thyroid dose to the population in the European Community varied somewhat because the levels of iodine contamination depended on the path of the radioactive plume and on the local climatic conditions. The thyroid dose received in the European Community during the first few weeks after the accident was almost entirely from ingestion of food stuffs, especially milk, contaminated by the radioactive iodine or by inhalation from the radioactive cloud. In general, parents in the more exposed areas avoided the use of fresh milk in the first weeks after the accident and the thyroid dose to children appears, over wide areas of the Community, to have been limited to an average of 3 to 10 mGray (mGy), and a thyroid dose about 5 to 10 times smaller for adults. For children, and for those exposed prenatally, the question of whether there would be a detectable increase in thyroid cancer in Western Europe was analyzed in detail. In December 1988, as part of the Post Chernobyl Activities, an International Panel of Independent Experts established by the Radiation Protection Programme drafted recommendations on the feasibility of carrying out studies on the health effects in Western Europe from environmental exposure to ionizing radiation as a consequence of the Chernobyl nuclear reactor accident (EUR 12551). After detailed analysis, the Panel concluded that there was no possible justification for thyroid studies in the European Community in connection with the reactor accident and the resulting radioactive contamination in the European countries. The experts concluded that any increased rates in thyroid cancer, even in those exposed prenatally or as children, will be so small as to remain undetectable.

If Western European children had received an average thyroid dose of 3 to 10 mGy, it seems that children who lived in the contaminated areas of Belarus and The Ukraine had received nearly a thousand times more with an average thyroid dose of 2 to 5 Gy and up to 1 Gy in Russia. These doses were estimated in May-June 1986 by the Institute of Biophysics, Moscow, based on measurements of thyroid radioactivity for 120,000 subjects, of which 30,000 were children, from the Belarus cities of Gomel and Minsk. To the best of our knowledge, radiation from short-lived isotopes was not adequately taken into account. An analysis of the data, which has never been released in full, showed that the largest thyroid exposure doses were received by children under 7 years of age who lived in the 30km zone at the time of the accident. The mean dose for this age group in the Khoiniki district was 5 Gy, for adults 1.5 Gy, and in Bragin 2 Gy for children of 0-7 years (data from the meeting in Minsk in October 1992). It is the opinion of the experts that we will never have completely accurate doses and these dose estimates must be considered to be approximate as, at present, there is no straightforward way to reconstruct the dose from internal emitters. At these high doses, (5 Gy total body dose is lethal) some effect on the thyroid of the children is to be anticipated as has been indicated in "The International Chernobyl - Technical Report" (IAEA, 1991). On the basis of the lifetime relative risk estimates defined for thyroid cancer by the International Commission for Radiological Protection in its Publication No.60 (ICRP, 1991) at a dose of 5 Gy to the childhood thyroid about 4000 thyroid cancers per 100,000 children exposed can be anticipated.

The reports of an increasing number of cases of childhood thyroid cancer in the years from 1986 to 1991 in the republic of Belarus first appeared in 1991. The number of reported cases has roughly doubled each year starting in 1988, and reached more than fifty per year in 1991 in a total population of 10 million adults and children. Recently an increase in thyroid cancer for the same age group of children has also been reported in the republic of Ukraine. This situation represents an important additional case load to the medical services responsible for diagnosis, treatment and follow-up, and it adds a severe burden to the lives of the directly affected children and their families.

These reports were treated initially with widespread scepticism by the scientific community but, in order to assess the validity of the claims of increased childhood thyroid cancer the Radiation Protection Research Action of the Commission of the European Community established a Panel of Thyroid Experts. Following a meeting of this panel in GSF Neuherberg in January 1992 and a consideration of pathological evidence in June 1992 the Panel visited Minsk in Belarus in October 1992 to examine, in collaboration with Belarussian physicians, the childhood thyroid cancer excess following the Chernobyl accident. One of the aims of the panel was to conduct a clinical examination of the patients, to look at the pathology of the cases,to examine case notes, to assess the data available thus far on thyroid cancer incidence, and to identify questions which still require carefully documented answers. During the one-week visit, the experts examined 26 young children who were either registered cases or suspected cases of thyroid cancer. Thyroid cancer in children is a rare disease worldwide, and the thyroid experts who make up this panel normally see only one or two children with thyroid cancer per year in their clinical practices so that the experience of seeing so many patients in one week was quite impressive.

As a consequence of the visit to Minsk, the examination of patients and patient data and participation in an international conference on Thyroid Cancer organised by the Ministry of Health of Belarus with the support of the World Health Organisation this panel has prepared a Consensus Opinion on the occurrence of childhood thyroid cancer in Belarus which is presented in this report. Independently of any further research on the incidence of childhood thyroid cancer in the three Republics, which is certainly required, the Panel considered that the present situation justified immediate action in relation to certain conclusions, and that much would be lost if this action was delayed.

The main aim of this report is therefore to document the situation as of November 1992, to formulate practical conclusions and draft recommendations in terms of public health and social policy, to ensure that opportunities to gain knowledge of the consequences of a major disaster are not lost, and moreover, in terms of clinical care, to help to ensure that the children presenting with thyroid tumours should receive the best possible medical attention. The international exchange of information on diagnostic and treatment methods and protocols already proposed by the "International Thyroid Associations" should be encouraged and used as a basis for advice on international assistance programmes.

5. The Thyroid, Iodine Isotopes and Cancer

5.1 Physiology of thyroid: role of iodine

The main function of the thyroid gland is to produce thyroid hormones, thyroxine (T4) and triiodothyronine (T3) which are essential to normal growth and development (Taurog, A., 1991). After manufacture, T4 and T3 are released from the gland into the blood to control oxidative processes in the tissues. Muscles, liver, heart, kidneys and virtually all the organs and systems of the body are affected by thyroid hormones. They play a fundamental role in the process of differentiation and maturation during embryonic and post-neonatal development. Thyroid activity is regulated by the thyroid-stimulating hormone (TSH) whose release by the pituitary is in turn dependent on the levels of circulating thyroid hormones. Secretion of TSH increases in response to a reduction of serum thyroid hormone concentrations, and the opposite occurs when thyroid hormones are augmented. Iodine is an essential substrate for the formation of thyroid hormones (Nagataki, S. & Ingbar, S.H., 1991). Normally, iodine is introduced through the diet and rapidly absorbed from the intestine as inorganic iodide. Inhalation and absorption through the skin and mucosa are usually negligible routes, but may be relevant under special circumstances (Briançon, C. et al., 1992). Serum iodide is concentrated by the thyroid gland through an active transport mechanism and incorporated in the protein thyroglobulin to form iodotyrosines, the precursors of thyroid hormones. Iodotyrosines are then coupled into T4 and T3 within the thyroglobulin molecule, and released after proteolysis into the blood, according to need, under the control of TSH. Thyroid hormones undergo metabolic processes leading to deiodination in peripheral tissues. Part of iodide resulting from this process is recovered directly by the thyroid gland. Iodide escaping thyroid uptake is largely excreted through the urine and, to a lesser extent, through the stools and sweat. Iodide crosses the placenta freely and is concentrated by the foetal thyroid gland beginning around the 12th week of gestation. Iodide is also concentrated in the lactating breast, both in humans and other mammals, and is secreted in the milk.

5.2 Iodine isotopes released in a nuclear accident

In the event of an accident in an operating nuclear reactor involving a release of radioactivity, the iodine isotopes will be among the first fission products to be released. Iodine, though a solid substance at room temperature, is volatile, and will be released in the form of a vapour in the elemental state at even slightly elevated temperatures. The Table below gives the nuclides of iodine, their half-lives and their relative abundance in the fission product mixture from a reactor operating at equilibrium. The relative abundance of the different isotopes is determined by a balance between the rate of production and the rate of decay so that for prompt events, such as a nuclear explosion, the short-lived nuclides are in greater relative abundance due solely to the rates of radioactive decay.

In addition to the isotopes of iodine themselves other fission products decay to yield radioactive isotopes of iodine, most notably isotopes of Xenon, a noble gas, and Tellurium-132. Tellurium, which is also a relatively volatile element from the same group

Table : Dosimetric data and resulting radiation doses for radio-iodines

	^{131}I	^{132}I	^{133}I	^{134}I	^{135}I	^{132}I associate with ^{132}Te
Radioactive half-life, T_r (days)	8.0	0.10	0.85	0.035	0.28	3.2
Effective half-life, T_{eff} (days) **child**	6.0	0.10	0.82	0.035	0.28	2.6
Effective half-life, T_{eff} (days) **adult**	7.6	0.10	0.84	0.035	0.28	2.6
Fraction to blood via inhalation, f_2	0.6	0.4	0.5	0.4	0.4	0.17
Effective fraction of activity from blood to thyroid, f_{eff} *child*	0.34	0.10	0.27	0.042	0.19	0.10
Effective fraction of activity from blood to thyroid, f_{eff} *adult*	0.29	0.09	0.23	0.036	0.16	0.09
Effective energy per disintegration, E (MeV)	0.2	0.4	0.45	0.45	0.3	0.4
Proportion of isotopes in fuel relative to Iodine-131*	1.0	1.2	1.8	2.2	1.7	1.2
Dose relative to that from Iodine-131	1.0	0.007	0.33	0.003	0.05	0.09

* Assuming equilibrium

of elements as sulphur, can enter the blood-stream through inhalation, and on decay to Iodine-132 leads to irradiation of the thyroid.

The routes of exposure to fallout radiation can be quite complex. External exposure can be received either from a passing fallout cloud or from immersion in it. Continued exposure during and after the passage of the cloud is likely from radionuclides deposited on the ground and buildings and internally from nuclides inhaled or ingested following their entry into the food chain. In the early phase of a release from an operating reactor significant external exposure may arise from the noble gases but their chemical inactivity means they are unlikely to lead to any significant internal exposure.

The isotopes of iodine are however metabolically active and once inhaled or ingested are retained in the thyroid. Their short radioactive half life (with the exception of Iodine-125, Iodine-129 and to a lesser extent Iodine-131) results in partial decay before the incorporation is complete thus somewhat reducing the dose. Neither do these very short-lived isotopes live long enough in general to enter the body by ingestion in food although exceptions may be water collected from the roofs of dwellings and milk consumed from privately owned cows, where in both cases the usual long period entailed in a distribution system is either short or non-existent.

For a given exposure which involves breathing contaminated air during the passage of the cloud and eating the food upon which deposition has taken place and drinking the milk from cows grazing the contaminated pastures the dominant route of entry for Iodine-131 is milk, inhalation accounting for only less than 10% of the total dose to the thyroid (Baverstock K.F., 1986). This assumes that milk is consumed until radioactive decay is effectively complete; if the milk supply is curtailed or inhabitants removed from the affected area then the components due to inhalation will assume a greater relative importance.

However, such conclusions are based on a number of assumed factors such as the breathing rate, which varies with the amount of exercise taken, the quantity of milk consumed each day, the access of cows to pasture etc. Deviations from these assumed parameters can markedly influence the projected doses and so it can be assumed that for individuals "reconstructed" doses are uncertain.

It is instructive to consider the relative contributions to thyroid dose from the external radiation associated with a fission product mix and that specifically from Iodine-131. Such an estimate can be obtained from the Chernobyl project report (IAEA International Chernobyl Project Technical Report, 1991). It can be shown that the contribution from I-131 to thyroid dose in infants, mainly due to consumption of contaminated milk in the month after the accident, can be as high as up to 50 times that from Cs isotopes (external and internal) during the four years after the accident. This is provided that controls on the level of Cs contamination in food are implemented in the long term in areas of heavy contamination and no prophylactic measures are taken to reduce iodine uptake, as was the case for most of the exposed populations around Chernobyl. Very close (within tens of km) to the site of the accident an additional component of external irradiation from immersion in the cloud of radioactive gases may apply.

5.3. Radiation induced thyroid cancer

The evidence that external radiation can be carcinogenic to the thyroid is overwhelming. The evidence that radiation to the thyroid from isotopes of iodine is carcinogenic to the human thyroid is less solid. External radiation to thyroid was first put forward as a cause of thyroid carcinoma in the 1950s when cases were found in children who had been treated by X-ray therapy in infancy for presumed enlarged thymus (Duffy and Fitzgerald, 1950). Numerous studies have been carried out since then, including very large cohort studies in the United States by Hempelmann and his colleagues (1975) using unirradiated siblings as controls for children who had received doses of several hundreds of rads, and in Israel by Ron and coworkers (1989) studying children given much smaller doses as part of the treatment of fungal infections. Radioactive isotopes of iodine have been used in man in several situations; they are given in extremely high doses in the treatment of thyroid cancer when the dose used is intended to kill all thyroid cells, subsequent thyroid cancers therefore do not arise. Isotopes of iodine are extensively used in the treatment of patients with thyrotoxicosis and in these circumstances there is no evidence of a subsequent excess incidence of thyroid cancers. Patients with thyrotoxicosis are very largely adults and their thyroid is in a very different physiological state from that of normal children. Small doses of isotopes of iodine have also been used in tracer studies of patients. Here there is again no convincing evidence of subsequent thyroid disorders. Many animal studies have shown that radioiodine is carcinogenic to the thyroid. Some of the earlier studies suggested that it was less effective than external radiation but one large recent study (Lee et al, 1982) found that in rats the carcinogenic potential of iodine 131 and X-rays were similar.

Human epidemiological experience has recently been reviewed by Shore (1992). The principal dose response relationship is probably linear and there is direct evidence to indicate a risk at low doses. Iodine 131 appears to be between 20 and 30% as effective as external X or gamma rays but there is little or no experience in young children. The dose rate may be important in the different carcinogenic potential. While the major increase in cases of thyroid cancer appears 10 to 15 years after exposure several studies have shown a small excess of thyroid cancer between 3 and 7 years after exposure. Both of the major types of differentiated thyroid carcinoma - papillary and follicular cancers - are caused by radiation; the risk of the development of papillary carcinoma is higher than that of follicular carcinoma.

In view of the lack of evidence on the carcinogenicity of iodine 131 in children and particularly in those with normally functioning thyroid it is generally assumed for radiological protection purposes that the risks associated with exposure to the isotopes of iodine are similar to those associated with exposure to external radiation. The International Committee for Radiation Protection has derived a life time risk factor for the radiation induction of fatal thyroid carcinoma in an exposed population of all ages of 0.08% per sievert. They also assume that the fatality rate for thyroid cancer will be 10% giving a life time risk of thyroid cancer incidence of 0.8% per sievert (Annals of ICRP 1991). These values are based on the NCRP report of 1985 and in view of the presumed linear nature of the dose response curve for external exposure are not adjusted for low doses.

A variety of factors other than radiation are important in the incidence of the three main types of thyroid carcinoma of follicular cell origin. These tumours are rare in infancy and childhood. Papillary and follicular carcinomas are much more common in women than in men although tumours in men are often more aggressive. Goitre and benign thyroid tumours are more common in iodine deficient areas. The relative prevalence of follicular and papillary thyroid carcinomas is dependent on iodine intake. Follicular carcinoma is more common in areas of iodine deficiency while papillary carcinoma is relatively more common in areas of iodine excess (Williams, 1985). Radiation is known to be a carcinogenic agent that can cause either papillary or follicular carcinoma with children being more susceptible than adults. Radiation may be one factor leading to the change from differentiated to undifferentiated carcinoma (Shimaoka, 1979).

Radiation is a mitogen, that is it causes damages to the DNA in a cell. When that damage is sufficiently severe the cell will die. When the damage is less severe the consequences will depend upon which genes are affected. The development of a cancer is thought to depend upon several DNA changes (mutations) in genes that control cell growth affecting one cell, with the mutations being acquired sequentially. In an over simplified and hypothetical example, mutation in gene A in one cell will give rise to a group of cells each affected by that mutation. One of these cells then acquires mutation in gene B, perhaps growing more rapidly to give a large group of cells, each bearing mutations in genes A and B. One of these cells in turn acquires mutation in gene C and a cell which bears mutations in genes A, B and C has the ability to invade and to give rise to distant metastases, so that its daughter cells form a cancer. Mutations can be caused by various chemicals and also by radiation. Work is currently in progress to attempt to link mutations to different causative agents. Some of the genes that show mutations are known for thyroid cancer and there are differences in the genes involved in the genesis of the three major types referred to above.

Interestingly, there is also evidence that follicular carcinoma may arise out of a preexisting benign tumour (follicular adenoma) while papillary carcinoma does not show any clearly defined change during progression from a microscopic lesion. Any factor leading to an increase in follicular carcinoma would be expected to be accompanied by an increase in follicular adenomas, the same is not true for factors that lead to an increase in papillary carcinoma.

In summary there is no doubt that thyroid cancer can be radiation induced. This has been conclusively shown for external radiation in man and animals and for radiation from isotopes of iodine in animals. The radioactive isotopes of iodine are mutagens that are selectively concentrated in the thyroid and it would be remarkable if they did not have a carcinogenic potential in man as they have in animals. Thyroid cancer has occurred in those exposed to fall-out from the Bravo nuclear test on northern atolls of the Marshall Islands. It must therefore be assumed that exposure to fall-out from a nuclear accident such as Chernobyl, particularly exposure of children , is likely to increase the incidence of thyroid cancer in the population. An increase between 3 and 5 years after exposure is unusual but not unprecedented and it is to be hoped that it does not serve as a pointer to a large and sustained increase in the years to come.

6. The reactor accident at Chernobyl and subsequent thyroid doses

The reactor accident

On April 26, 1986, at 01.23 (Moscow time) the reactor operators lost control of the number four unit of the Chernobyl nuclear power station; the reactor went from a very low power level into a power surge, exploded and caught fire. The explosion ejected large amounts of radioactive debris into the atmosphere and the fire melted the fuel elements in the core of the reactor, releasing the more volatile radioactive fission products and the radioactive fission product noble gases such as krypton and xenon.

The reactor was being closed down after a considerable period of operation at full power but was held, with increasing difficulty, at very low power in order to make a specific test, when it got out of control. The radioactive inventory of the core of the reactor at the time of the accident has been estimated to be 40×10^{18} Becquerel (Bq) (10^9 Curie (Ci)) and some 4% of the total activity of the core of the reactor is thought to have escaped into the atmosphere in the ten days following the explosion before the releases were finally curtailed (IAEA, 1991). The major emission of about 25% of the total radioactivity released in the accident occurred immediately after the explosion and was considerably decreased on days 2 to 6 after the accident by preventative activities of emergency workers. On day 7 omissions again started to increase with a second peak of emission on days 9 and 10. During days 2 to 6 attempts were made to cool the damaged core of the reactor by dropping boron, dolomite, sand, clay and lead on to it from helicopters, and the radioactive release was mainly from finely dispersed uranium fuel particles. However, in the period from 7 to 10 days after the accident the core temperature increased and a second wave of volatile fission products was emitted, including iodine. The radioactive debris and larger fuel particles were deposited in the region near to the reactor but finer fuel particles and the volatile fission products spread further and contamination from the accident was detected in most of western Europe.

The radioactive plume

Although only about 4% of the total core activity is thought to have escaped, 100% of the noble gases krypton and xenon and 15 - 20% of the tellurium and iodine activities of the core are considered to have been released (IAEA, 1991). There are, however, other estimates of amounts of activity released giving different percentages such as 100% of the noble gases, 10% of the tellurium, 60% of the iodine and 40% of the caesium (Gudiksen et al., 1991). It needs to be emphasized that these estimates of released radioactivity are approximate and the true amount of emitted radioactivity still remains to be established. According to the Technical Report of the International Chernobyl Project published by the International Atomic Energy Agency in 1991, some 3.3×10^{16} Bq of Krypton-85, 1.7×10^{18} Bq of Xenon-133, 2.6×10^{17} Bq of Iodine-131 and 5×10^{16} Bq of Tellurium-132 as well as 2×10^{16} Bq of Caesium-134 and 3×10^{16} Bq of Caesium-137 were released into the atmosphere in the explosion and fire. In the first 24 hours the ratio of Iodine to Caesium was 22:1, and this decreased to 8:1 after 48 hours and to 5:1 in the period from 3 to 5 days after the accident.

Meteorology

The weather at the time of the accident was calm with light, variable winds and the cloud of radioactivity drifted West and North over Northern Ukraine and Southern Belarus. At higher altitudes there was a stronger wind from the south-east which was responsible for carrying radioactivity as far as Sweden where it was first detected on April 27. The majority of the radioactivity released did not rise above 600m although some activity was found in the first two days up to an altitude of 1800m. On April 29, the wind direction changed and the cloud moved eastward and then, on April 30, southwards. The low wind speed, the variable direction of the wind and very local rain showers led to a variable level of contamination over wide areas of Northern Ukraine, Southern and Western Belarus and the Briansk and Kaluga regions of Russia which border Northern Ukraine and Southern Belarus, with some local high levels of contamination resulting from the local rain showers.

The most important element from the point of view of thyroid cancer is iodine which is taken up and concentrated in the thyroid gland and in this respect it is important to realise that Xenon-133 decays, with a half-life of 5.27 days, to Iodine-133 which has a half-life of 0.85 days, and that Tellurium-132 decays, with a half-life of 3 days, to Iodine-132, which has a half-life of 0.10 days. Thus, in addition to the Iodine 131, with a half-life of 8.05 days, there was probably a considerable amount of shorter lived isotopes of Iodine in the cloud of released radioactivity. Until now no good estimates of iodine contamination, especially of the short lived isotopes, of the areas around Chernobyl are available but it is clear that the contamination maps of Caesium-137 cannot be used to predict completely the contamination of iodine. However, it must be anticipated that the local variations in the deposition level of Caesium-137 which can still be found imply that the contamination of iodine was also subject to strong local fluctuations dependent on local weather conditions.

The life-style of the population

Northern Ukraine, Southern Belarus and the Briansk and Kaluga regions of Russia which were most contaminated by the radioactive plume are predominantly agricultural areas with many small settlements and few major towns, of which Gomel in Belarus, Novozybkov in the Briansk region of Russia and Ovruch and Korosten in the Northern Ukraine are examples. The major cities of Kiev and Minsk were also contaminated, Minsk more so than Kiev, but to a lesser extent than the towns closer to the reactor and more directly in the path of the radioactive plume. The populations living in the areas north and west of the reactor are mainly involved in low quality agriculture, because of the poor soils, and forestry. They live in simple houses and spend much of the time out of doors, in warm weather many children sleep outside and many families own their own "private" cow and grow their own vegetables. Much of the soil is sandy with some peat soils and marshland, they have a low natural fertility and are poor in mineral nutrients. The whole area is low in natural iodine salts and is recognized as an area of mild endemic goitre. In the late 1970's the diet of the population had been supplemented with iodine to reduce the incidence of goitre but in the early 1980's, and certainly by 1985, this practice had fallen into abeyance. The low level of natural iodine in the general diet meant that any additional exposure, for instance to radioactive iodine, would be likely to result in a rapid and near complete uptake into the thyroid. An intense uptake of radioactive iodine leads to high radiation doses to the thyroid of both adults and, especially, children because the relative concentration of radioactivity per unit mass of thyroid is higher in the smaller thyroids of the children. One method to prevent the intense uptake of radioactive iodine into the thyroid is to block the thyroid with stable iodine, usually by taking potassium iodide tablets.

This form of prophylaxis is well known and recommended as an immediate preventive measure in the case of a nuclear accident. However, although there are reports of the wide scale distribution of potassium iodide in affected regions, in Belarus, at least, very little indication of its use was revealed from conversations between Panel members and scientists and doctors in the republic. If stable iodine was available and distributed to the population in the affected areas it seems likely that it was distributed too late to have had any prophylactic effect for those living in northern Ukraine and southern Belarus who were exposed to the first plume of radioactivity.

In the first few days after the accident the population was not told about the accident but learnt about it from those who were recruited as drivers to evacuate people on April 27 from the town of Pripyat, situated very close to the reactor. Those who did learn about the accident in this way did not realize how serious the situation was and that they might also be affected by it. On April 28 people and cattle were evacuated from a zone of 10km radius around the reactor and on May 2, the decision was taken to evacuate people from a zone of 30km radius around the reactor; this was completed by May 6. General information on the accident seems to have been made available officially for the first time some 3 to 4 days after the accident but it is not clear whether the people were told about preventive measures to be taken to reduce exposure. Some people seem to have taken simple preventive measures like remaining indoors, taking iodine compounds, not drinking milk or eating fresh vegetables, but others did not take any steps to prevent or limit their exposure to the radioactivity.

The delay in informing the population about the accident, the obvious lack of any form of prophylaxis during the first few days, and the variable response of the population to the information of the accident together with the propensity of the population to "live off the land" consuming fresh milk and vegetables, and the variable levels of contamination as a result of local weather conditions, resulted in a very large population being exposed to high levels of radioactive iodine with consequently high radiation doses to their thyroid glands.

Thyroid doses

The radiation exposure of the population living in the path of the radioactive plume was both external, such as radiation emitted by the radioactive cloud or from radioactivity deposited on the ground, and from internal radioactivity that was ingested or inhaled, both pathways being important in the first few days after the accident. The initial evacuation measures were taken on the basis of estimates of accumulated total body dose from external radiation so that the level of dose was limited, by the evacuation, to well below that at which any indication of acute effects of radiation are expected. The dose to the thyroid glands of the population from external radiation is therefore unlikely to have been significant. However, the thyroid gland concentrates any iodine which is inhaled and taken up in the blood or ingested in food, especially when the level of natural iodine in the diet is low. The concentration of radioactive iodine in the thyroid means that the dose of radiation to the thyroid can be disproportionately high compared with a total body dose, and because radiation dose is defined as the amount of energy deposited in tissue per unit weight of tissue, the same amount of radioactive iodine concentrated in smaller thyroid glands gives a proportionally higher dose to the thyroid. This means that in the situation occurring after the accident when both young children and adults were exposed to similar levels of radioactive iodine, the dose to the thyroid gland of the children was five to ten times greater than the dose to the adult thyroid. It should also be remembered that the thyroid gland first starts to take up iodine when the foetus is about 12 weeks old and that radioactive iodine will pass from the mothers blood to the foetal blood, so that exposure of the mother to radioiodine after the 12th week of pregnancy will result in concentration of radioiodine by the foetal thyroid. Radioiodine is also concentrated in human breast milk, so that mothers exposed to fallout will pass relatively high concentrations of radioactive iodine to babies being breastfed.

The doses which have been estimated for the population of the affected areas are based on measurements of thyroid activities using both specially designed and calibrated detectors and other more general detection equipment. These thyroid measurements, made on a large number of people hopefully giving a good cross-section of the affected population, first started on May 6, ten days after the accident, and are therefore essentially based on the contamination by Iodine-131, the longest lived of the important radioactive iodine isotope fission products. An estimate of the accumulated dose to the thyroid is based on a calculation which takes account of the decay of the isotope with a physical half-life of 8.05 days and some assumptions about the biological half-life for the retention of iodine in the thyroid, the pattern of uptake in the period from April 26 and the date of the measurements. The proportion of short-lived isotopes of iodine should also be taken into account. Some 250,000 measurements of thyroid activity in Belarus were made after the accident, although many of these measurements were made with less reliable equipment than that available in the Ukraine. The Institute of Biophysics in Moscow has been concerned with converting these measurements to dose but full details of actual dose estimates have not are currently been made available. Very few actual measurements of the short lived isotopes of iodine can have been made and the dose to the thyroid caused by these short lived isotopes cannot be considered to have been determined directly. It is probable that the most important exposure pathway for the short lived iodine isotopes was via inhalation from the cloud and it will be extremely difficult, if not impossible, to estimate the contribution of dose to the thyroid from this pathway. Even so, it has to be borne in mind that in certain parts of Western Europe, Sweden, Germany and the Netherlands (Arntsing et al., 1991; CEC Contractors Meeting, 1986; Stoutjesdijk & Zoeteman, 1987), measurements of radioactive contamination from the Chernobyl accident registered comparable levels of Tellurium-132 and Iodine-131 activity about one week after the accident which suggests that there could have been a considerably important level of short lived iodine isotopes in the first plume. However, the most important pathway for radioactive iodine exposure to the thyroid is considered to be via food and especially via milk, so that those people with their own cow who continued to drink the milk after the accident were probably at the greatest risk.

The dose calculations which have been made suggest that the doses to the children's thyroids in parts of Southern Belarus were of the order of several Gy, with 1% of children having doses above 10 Gy accumulated chronically over several days (for comparison, a total-body dose of 5 Gy accumulated acutely will give an acute radiation syndrome and can be lethal). The chronic accumulation of the thyroid dose will certainly lead to a reduced effect compared to an acute dose, accumulated over 1 or 2 hours, but even so these doses to the children's thyroids have to be considered as abnormally high and potentially dangerous doses. These doses are subject to considerable error and could underestimate the true dose because of the uncertainty about the contribution of the short lived isotopes of iodine to this dose. Thus, it will be extremely difficult ever to determine the thyroid doses to the children with any degree of confidence unless new techniques of retrospective dosimetry become available. One possibility is that cytological dosimetry can be developed to provide measurements of the thyroid tissue which will give a more direct measure of accumulated dose. The doses to the adult thyroid will, in general, be an order of magnitude lower than those in the children and there is therefore a lower probability for an effect.

Current radiological protection philosophy assumes that the probability for the induction of malignancy by radiation increases in direct proportion with the dose, especially when the dose is accumulated chronically. Thus, this philosophy predicts that the younger children who accumulated the highest thyroid doses are at the highest risk of developing thyroid cancer, and while it cannot be denied that there are probably other factors which can influence the magnitude of this risk it would be unrealistic, in view of the level of the doses accumulated, not to anticipate the occurrence of some childhood thyroid cancers.

It is important to realize that the release of radioactive iodine from the reactor was greatest in the early days, but continued for up to about 10 days. Ten half lives of iodine 131 later the level of exposure will have dropped to less than one thousandth of the original levels, i.e. less than 12 weeks. The fetal thyroid does not concentrate radioiodine before 12 weeks of gestation. Putting these facts together it can be seen that children conceived before the end of January 1986 are at risk of exposure to radioiodine, that risk declines rapidly with later conceptions, and becomes negligible for children conceived after April 1986.

Children in Belarus are defined as under 15 years of age, and the incidence of thyroid cancer in the group is expected to decline with time as the exposed cohorts are replaced by unexposed cohorts. It is difficult to be certain whether the increased risk of thyroid cancer in the children exposed to radiation from isotopes of iodine at young ages will continue as these children become adults. It is even more difficult to estimate what the risk for thyroid cancer is for the population who were exposed as adults and who may have received thyroid doses of about 1 Gy. The evidence from children exposed to external radiation suggests that the increased risk of developing thyroid cancer will be retained through adolescence and for many years of adulthood.

7. Thyroid Cancer in Children after the Chernobyl accident

7.1. Present Evidence Related to Chernobyl

The phenomenon of childhood thyroid cancer following the Chernobyl nuclear accident can be examined in terms of the observed increase in incidence rates, the geographic distribution of increased rates, the effect of screening on observed incidence rates and the clinical and histopathological nature of the observed tumours. So far, increases of childhood thyroid cancer incidence rates have been reported from the republics of the Belarus and Ukraine, but not from the Russian republic. Data from the Ukraine have not yet been reported in detail and, at this time, the best organized data sources are those from the republic of Belarus, from where the following data are taken (Abelin et al., 1993).

7.1.a. Increase of childhood thyroid cancer incidence rates

An increase of disease incidence rates can be compared both with rates observed elsewhere in the world and in terms of trends observed within exposed regions. In the republic of Belarus, which has a well developed cancer registry, there was an increase in the rates of confirmed cases of thyroid cancer among children aged 0-14 years as follows:

- 1978-1988   :   between 0 and 0.14/100,000/yr.

- 1989:   :   0.25/100,000/yr (confirmed cases)

- 1990   :   1.15/100,000/yr. (confirmed cases)

- 1991   :   2.25/100,000/yr.

The increase was about twenty-fold from before the accident to 1991 for the whole of Belarus. A review of "Cancer Incidence on Five Continents" (Muir et al., 1987) and a recalculation of rates shows that the average yearly childhood thyroid cancer incidence rate for the combination of the cancer registries of four Nordic countries (Denmark, (1978-82), Finland (1977-81), Norway (1978-82) and Sweden (1978-82)) was 0.1/100,000 yr.; for the combination of four Eastern European cancer registries (Cracow, Poland (1978-81), Nowy Sacz, Poland (1978-81), Warsaw City (1980-82) and Slovakia (1978-82)) it was 0.04/100,000/yr., and rates for the largest cancer registries in the United States reached 0.3/100,000/yr. (McWriter & Petroeschevsky, 1990). These rates are consistent with those reported within Belarus up to 1988 and suggest case registration in Belarus to be comparable to other cancer registries.

7.1.b.   Geographic distribution of increased rates

As the following table shows, incidence rates of 1991 childhood thyroid cancer differed greatly within Belarus, with definitely the highest rates in the Gomel region, closest to Chernobyl:

<u>Oblast (Region)</u>	<u>Rate per 100,000/yr.</u>
Gomel	9.6
Brest	1.1
Minsk county	0.8
Minsk city	0.5
Grodno	1.1
Mogilev	1.0
Vitebsk	0.3

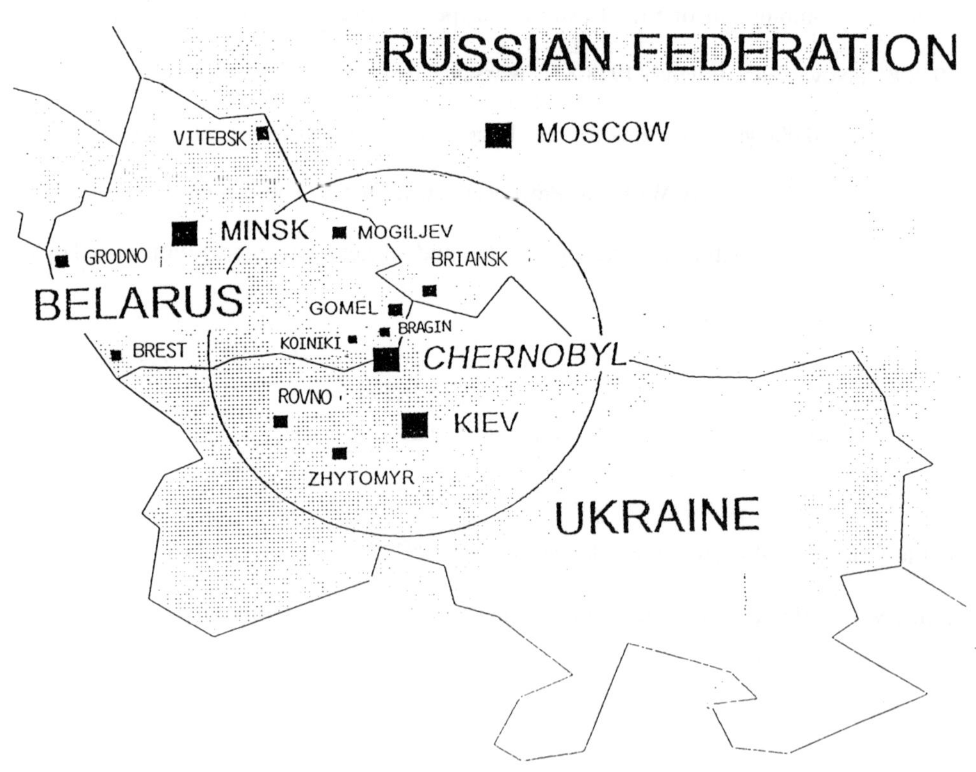

An analysis by districts (Rayons) within Gomel Oblast for 1990 and 1991 combined shows that again, the area closest to the Chernobyl accident site (districts of Narovlia, Koiniki, Bragin, Loev combined) had the highest rate (13.1.), followed by Gomel city (8.4) and the other areas of the Oblast (2.7 to 5.4 for different groups of districts).

All cases (100%) reported from the four districts named above as being closest to the accident site and from the four western-most districts of Gomel Oblast had tumours that were at least 15mm in diameter and/or had developed lymph node metastases, whereas this was the case in only 63 to 75 percent of the cases reported from the other areas. This could be interpreted to suggest a certain effect of active case finding on the stage at tumour detection in the areas further away from Chernobyl and thus less exposed to Iodine-131.

TABLE

Distribution of confirmed cases of thyroid cancer by age at exposure, age at diagnosis and sex, Belarus, 1986-1991

Year at diagnosis	Age at exposure (years)			Age at diagnosis (years)			Sex	
	0-4	5-9	10-14	0-4	5-9	10-14	M	F
1986	-	-	1	-	-	1	-	1
1987	-	-	-	-	-	-	-	-
1988	-	2	1	-	2	1	1	2
1989	1	4	1	1	1	4	4	2
1990	12	8	3	2	15	6	13	10
1991	31	22	-*	-	31	22	19	34
Total	44	36	6	3	49	34	37	49

* no cases in this group possible in 1991

Of the 86 histologically verified cases occurring between 1986 and 1991, more than half of the cases were between 0 and 4 years old at the time of the accident and many of the rest were 5 to 9 years old. At diagnosis more than half of the cases were between 5 and 9 years old and many of the rest were between 10 and 14 years old. This data indicates that the first cancers are starting to appear after about 4 years, in accordance with what has been found previously for childhood thyroid cancer.

It should be noted that as time passes the cohort of children in the 10 - 14 year age group at the time of the accident will gradually decrease as these children move into the group above 15 years of age and are classified as young adults and in 1991 this cohort would be zero. Cancers arising in this group after they had turned 15 would no longer be classified as childhood cancers. Unfortunately no information is as present available to us on the occurrence of thyroid cancer in young adults in Belarus.

Similarly, the low number of cases noted in the 0 - 4 year group at diagnosis is not surprising as this cohort contains a decreasing proportion of children who were actually exposed to radioactive iodine from the Chernobyl accident as the year at diagnosis increases. The number of cases is further decreased by the latency period between exposure and the appearance of the tumour which seems to be at least 3 years.

In fact, if the radioactive iodine exposure from the Chernobyl accident is the cause of the thyroid cancers then there should be a sharp drop in the cancer incidence in children who were conceived after April 1986 and whose thyroids were unaffected by the radioactive iodine compared with those children who were born before the accident. A study of the cancer incidence in children as a function of date of birth through the period of the accident could provide the best indication of whether the Chernobyl accident is indeed the cause of the childhood thyroid cancers.

7.1.c.   The impact of screening on case ascertainment

The confirmation of the pathological diagnosis of thyroid carcinoma in children in Belarus removes one of the obstacles to accepting the claim that a great increase in incidence of this tumour has occurred, starting about four years after the Chernobyl accident. The second major concern has been the possibility that the true frequency of this tumour has not changed, but that many more cases have come to light because of the screening programmes that have been undertaken or because general increased awareness and concern has led to more cases coming to medical attention.

For increased ascertainment to be a major cause implies that there is a reservoir of undiagnosed cases of thyroid cancer in the population, either cases that would never present or cases that present earlier than would otherwise be the case. Papillary thyroid carcinoma is normally a slowly growing disease and studies of autopsy thyroids have shown that undiagnosed carcinomas are relatively common. These tumours, however, are less than 1.0 cm in diameter, often only a few millimetres across or less and as their older name of occult carcinoma implies are usually clinically impalpable. They might therefore be detected by sensitive ultrasound techniques, but would not be found by clinical examination or observed as a swelling by concerned relatives. While they are common in adults they are much less common in young children (Franssilla and Harach, 1986).

When screening for thyroid carcinoma was introduced in Chicago for adults who had been irradiated in childhood an approximately 8 fold increase in the incidence of thyroid carcinoma was found (Ron et al, 1992). The tumours discovered by screening, however, showed a considerable reduction in median size and an approximately four fold increase in the proportion of tumours that were "microscopic" (Schneider et al, 1985). In contrast in Southern Belarus the increase in incidence of childhood thyroid cancer is calculated as approximately 80 fold. As these are children any reservoir of undiagnosed disease will be less than in adults. Small intrathyroid cancers were infrequent in the Belarus series and over half the cases showed direct extra thyroid extension. These therefore represent clinically significant disease, not occult cancers. It is therefore unlikely that they have been found because of concern about the effects of Chernobyl, and would not otherwise have presented. In the group of children seen by members of the EC mission over half had presented by non-screening routes.

Screening is necessary in an attempt to improve treatment of the disease but it will make it more difficult to assess the true size of the outbreak unless it is carried out at the same intensity in an unexposed group. As it becomes more effective and widely used it will hopefully pick up cases at a stage before normal clinical presentation and allow effective early therapy. The influence of screening on the apparent frequency of thyroid carcinoma in children in Belarus must be carefully considered in assessing the results but there is no evidence to show that it alone can explain the size of the present increase in incidence of childhood thyroid cancer.

7.2 Pathology confirmation

The reported increase in incidence of thyroid carcinoma in children in Belarus is an observation of very considerable importance. An essential component of the verification of this observation is the study of the pathology of the lesions. It is necessary to classify the tumours using internationally accepted criteria and to document features that may be relevant to the interpretation of the findings.

The classification of the pathology of thyroid tumours that is now widely used internationally is that of the World Health Organization (Hedinger et al, 1980). Malignant tumours may be derived from any of the four cell types that are normally found in the thyroid. These are the follicular cells, C cells, lymphoid cells and connective tissue cells. The great majority of the naturally occurring tumours are of follicular cell origin and these are the only group where radiation has been convincingly shown to be carcinogenic. Carcinomas of follicular cell origin include two major types of well differentiated carcinoma (papillary and follicular) and one type of undifferentiated carcinoma which may arise by progression from either of the differentiated carcinomas. Carcinomas of C cell origin are known as medullary carcinomas; about 20% of these tumours arise as a consequence of an inherited predisposition. Malignant lymphomas are related to autoimmune disease of the thyroid; tumours of connective tissue are very rare. It should be noted that the terms papillary and follicular can be used as either descriptive of the tissue architecture or as diagnostic terms, describing types of cancer, each characterised by a constellation of features, not just tissue architecture. A papillary carcinoma often contains some follicular elements and is occasionally dominated by cells with a follicular architecture.

The World Health Organization classification was used in the analyses of the tumours from Belarus. These tumours were originally diagnosed by Belarussian pathologists, and the great majority of their diagnoses were confirmed when they were re-examined by visiting Western pathologists. Initially, 93 cases diagnosed as thyroid cancer in Belarussian children under the age of 15 who had been operated on between 1986 and 1991 were reviewed by *Professor B. Egloff* and *Dr. C. Ruchti* of Switzerland. Eight further cases from that time period were unavailable. Later, 25 cases from 1992 were reviewed by *Professor E. D. Williams* from the United Kingdom and a further 17 by *Professor B. Egloff,* giving an overall total of 135 cases examined by independent expert pathologists.

Analysis of the 93 cases has been completed (Furmanchuk et al, 1992). The diagnosis of malignancy was confirmed in 86 (92.5%), 83 were clearly papillary carcinomas, and 3 were probable papillary carcinomas. The reason for the lack of confirmation of the diagnosis in 7 cases was in part inadequate material available for study and they were regarded as of doubtful malignancy. The 83 papillary carcinomas showed either areas of papillary structure, or, if dominated by follicular architecture, showed the nuclear changes and lack of encapsulation typical of papillary carcinoma. None showed the features of follicular, medullary or anaplastic carcinomas. Many of the tumours showed extensive fibrosis and abundant psammoma bodies, again features of papillary carcinoma. The presence of solid epithelial areas was common in these tumours although it is an unusual feature in papillary carcinoma in adults. The level of differentiation of tumours was classified according to the criteria proposed by Tscholl-Ducommun and Hedinger (1982), based on the extent of the solid areas. Of the 83 clear cut papillary carcinomas grading was not possible in one case, 18 showed the features of the follicular variant of papillary carcinoma. Only 13 were the typical, well differentiated papillary carcinoma commonly seen in adults, the remainder being classified as moderately or poorly differentiated.

During examination of the histological sections, extension of the tumour through the capsule was recorded, when present, together with any vascular invasion and any involvement of lymph nodes by the tumour. Fresh or fixed surgical material was not available for re-examination, only the histological slides. The clinical data from the operation was incorporated together with the histological observations to determine the staging of the tumours shown in the accompanying table.

Size of Primary tumour (T)		Lymph nodes		Distant metastases	
T1 (<1cm) 10	(11.5%)	2/10	(20%)	0	
T2 (1-4cm) 19	(22%)	12/19	(63%)	0	
T3 (>4cm) 3	(3.5%)	1/3	(33.3%)	0	
T4[1] 52	(60.5%)	45/52	(86.5%)	3	(6%)
TX[2] 2	(2.5%)	---		---	

At follow-up, 4 more cases showed lymph node metastases and another 3 cases had developed distant metastases. All distant metastases were lung metastases. One child

---

[1]T4: Extending to surrounding tissue

[2]TX: Size unknown

was reported to have died of widespread tumour, and macroscopic examination of the post mortem lungs showed very numerous relatively small grey tumour deposits throughout the parenchyma. A striking feature of many of these tumours is the aggressiveness, with vascular invasion and capsular penetration in small primary tumours. Tumours with direct extra thyroid extension would sometimes measure not more than 1.5 cm in diameter.

Of the 86 patients, 49 were girls with a female to male ratio of 1.3:1. The mean age of patients was 9.0 years at the time of diagnosis and 4.6 years at the time of the nuclear accident. 93% of the patients were younger than 9 years at the time of the accident. The mean interval between accident and diagnosis of cancer was 4.4 years. The examination of the additional cases once more confirmed the diagnoses made in Belarus. One was a medullary carcinoma which had been confirmed immunochemically, the remainder were again papillary carcinomas, showing essentially the same features as the previous series.

The observations leave no doubt that a large number of children have had thyroid carcinomas resected in Belarus in the years 1986-1992. The diagnoses made have been confirmed by independent observers and the tumours classified according to WHO criteria. The tumours are nearly all papillary carcinomas, and a considerable proportion show direct invasion of extrathyroid tissues. The pathological characteristics of the tumours are similar to those reported for other series of thyroid carcinoma in children (Schlumberger, 1987; Ceccarelli et al., 1988). The diagnoses of 76 thyroid carcinomas in children aged 15 or less were confirmed in Minsk in the 2 years 1990 to 1991. Minsk is the main centre for thyroid surgery in Belarus, with a population of about 10 million, but a high proportion of the children come from the Southern part of the country which has a population of about 2 million.

The Panel members had the opportunity to examine personally 26 children who were either registered cases or suspect cases of thyroid cancer. Results of diagnostic procedures on these subjects including haematological and biochemical data, were analysed and discussed with local physicians. Chest X-rays from the 3 children with lung metastases were also examined. There was a substantial agreement on the diagnosis of virtually all cases between the Panel members and the Belarussian physicians. In addition, the clinical records of 34 confirmed cases of thyroid cancer in children were made available for review. The overall impression of the Panel was that in most cases the clinical and laboratory features were in keeping with those expected in childhood thyroid cancer, including a high prevalence of lymph node metastases at diagnosis (Schlumberger et al., 1987; Ceccarelli et al., 1988).

The following facts serve to put these numbers in context; at the Institute Gustave-Roussy in Paris, an Institute with a major interest and international reputation in thyroid carcinoma which draws its patients from a very wide area of Europe, 72 thyroid carcinomas in children aged 16 or less have been treated in the period from 1945 - 1985 (Schlumberger, 1987). These 72 cases treated in France were accumulated over 40 years, while 76 Belarussian cases have occurred in 2 years. This comparison supports the conclusion that an unusually high level of childhood thyroid cancer has been recorded in Belarus since the Chernobyl accident. Obviously, careful epidemiological studies are needed to determine the true extent of the increase in incidence of childhood thyroid carcinoma in Belarus which must be based on carefully verified pathological diagnoses. This basis is now available.

The unique nature of the Chernobyl event and the obvious assumption that the high numbers of thyroid cancer might be associated with exposure to the radioactive iodine released in the accident requires that work be undertaken to investigate the relationship between thyroid carcinoma and the causative event. It is likely that the pattern of molecular biological defects differs between tumours, depending on the mutagenic agent involved, and studies are needed to compare the type and frequency of specific oncogene mutations in the childhood tumours found in the neighbourhood of Chernobyl with spontaneous tumours coming from other parts of Europe. These mutagenic changes should be compared to those found in human tumours known to be radiation induced from other sources, and must be carefully considered together with expert morphological description, and with other studies using immunohistochemistry and in situ hybridization to detect differentiation markers and oncogene products.

It is important to create a tissue bank of thyroid tumours and normal tissues from the Chernobyl regions, both fresh and fixed material, and to study cytogenetic changes in the tumours, including chromosomal breaks, loss of heterozygosity, translocations, and specific aberrations. Indeed, a study of the cytological state of non-neoplastic thyroid tissue from cancer cases may be an indirect way of assessing the radiation dose to the thyroids.

The epidemiology which is critical to an understanding of the exact relationship between the occurrence of thyroid cancer and the causative event, itself depends on the methods of ascertainment and on the accuracy of pathological diagnosis. The accuracy of diagnosis made in Minsk has been largely confirmed - but the two-tier method of ascertainment and diagnosis of thyroid carcinomas in Belarus, by which all tumours suspected of being malignant are referred to and operated on in Minsk while tumours thought to be benign are operated locally (periphery and Minsk), is complex, and no external assessment has been made by the Panel of the diagnoses made outside Minsk. Studies are required of the pathology of tumours removed peripherally but not referred to Minsk for confirmation of diagnosis. Pathological study of the material is essential for completeness and accuracy of the assessment of the numbers of thyroid carcinomas on which the epidemiology must be based. In addition, this material can be used for molecular biological studies and other work.

8. Prevention, diagnosis and management of disease

Prevention

Measures to be considered for the prevention of the development of thyroid cancer and other thyroid disorders in a radiation-exposed population include correction of iodine deficiency (if present) by iodine prophylaxis, and suppression of TSH by administration of thyroid hormones. The rationale for such measures is as follows:

a)   Dietary iodine deficiency is the major cause of endemic goitre and may result in a number of other disorders, including hypothyroidism, cretinism and various neurological defects. The question of whether and to what extent iodine deficiency *per se* also affects the development of thyroid cancer has been a matter of controversy. But evidence to date strongly suggests that the secondary rise in TSH in iodine deficiency is a factor in thyroid carcinogenesis.

An increased prevalence of thyroid cancer as a whole has been reported in some (Belfiore et al., 1987) but not (Ramalingaswami et al., 1969) all endemic goitre regions (Lindsay et al., 1966). More commonly, an increased proportion of the more aggressive type of differentiated thyroid cancer, follicular carcinoma, has been observed in iodine-deficient areas, a shift from follicular to papillary thyroid carcinoma occurring after effective iodine prophylaxis (Williams E D, 1985). Experimental data indicate that iodine deficiency favours the induction of thyroid neoplasms in animals exposed to thyroid irradiation (Lindsay et al, 1961).

Thus, correction of iodine deficiency by supplementation of dietary iodine with iodized salt or iodide tablets may contribute to the reduction of the incidence of thyroid carcinoma in irradiated subjects.

b)   Chronic thyroid stimulation by TSH leads to development of thyroid nodules and may favour the development of thyroid carcinoma. Experimental work indicates that increased thyroid stimulation, whether induced by iodine deficiency or thyroid blockade, is a factor in the carcinogenetic effect of thyroid irradiation (Williams E D, 1981). Hypothyroidism can also result from radiation, both external and internal. Evidence that this may occur after environmental exposure to radioisotopes of iodine was provided by the study of the Marshall islands population exposed to fallout. In this case hypothyroidism was apparently unrelated to thyroid autoimmunity, but an increased prevalence of autoimmune thyroiditis with thyroid insufficiency was observed in the survivals of the Hiroshima and Nagasaki atomic bomb explosions. The sustained increase in TSH secretion resulting from radiation-induced hypothyroidism might contribute to thyroid tumorigenesis. Once developed, differentiated thyroid cancer retains a number of biological functions of the normal thyroid, including TSH dependency.

Thus, suppression of TSH by the administration of thyroxine may be considered as an additional preventive measure. However, administration of suppressive doses of thyroxine is not without risk, especially in children, and requires careful monitoring to avoid iatrogenic thyrotoxicosis. This is clearly difficult to manage (if not impossible) as well as expensive, if applied to the entire irradiated population. On a cost/benefit basis this type of prophylactic thyroid suppressive therapy may be recommended only in irradiated subjects with proven thyroid lesions.

Considerable parts of Belarus, Ukraine and Russia are iodine deficient. Iodine prophylaxis was established in Belarus several years ago, but, unfortunately, was discontinued shortly before the Chernobyl accident. This may have adversely influenced thyroid irradiation by increasing the thyroidal uptake of radioiodine isotopes released by the nuclear reactor. Admittedly, iodine prophylaxis would have been much more efficient if operative before the accident; however, it may well be advantageous by reducing the late carcinogenetic effects of radiation. A side benefit of iodine prophylaxis would be to decrease markedly the incidence of goitre and especially nodular goitre in the population.

Diagnosis

Ultrasound imaging with transducers of at least 7.5 MHz used by well trained operators is the method of choice to study the morphology of the thyroid in children. Nodules or focal lesions as small as 5mm in diameter can be visualized and cystic nodules differentiated from solid nodules which carry a greater risk of thyroid cancer. Enlarged neck lymph nodes may also be localized.

The use of thyroid scanning with either 131-I or Tc^{99m} provides additional functional and morphological information. However, the use of thyroid scanning is not indicated for mass screening purposes, but it is useful for the differentiation of functioning (hot, i.e.

concentrating radioactive tracer) from non-functioning (cold) thyroid nodules. Malignant thyroid lesions are almost exclusively found in cold nodules. Neither thyroid ultrasonography nor scanning are sufficient to differentiate with certainty between benign and malignant thyroid nodules. Fine needle aspiration cytology of all cold nodules is mandatory for a reliable diagnosis. With experience, a correct preoperative diagnosis of malignancy can be established in most cases, with a sensitivity and specificity of more than 90%.

Ultrasound imaging is currently being carried out in several centres in Belarus and other CIS countries, using adequate modern equipment. Thyroid scanning is not used in Belarus because of the lack of appropriate facilities. Fine needle aspiration is performed by skilled personnel in major referral centres.

Therapy

Total or near-total thyroidectomy is commonly regarded in the West as the treatment of choice, since thyroid cancer in children after exposure to radiation often shows multifocal growth and invasion beyond the thyroid capsule (up to 50% of the cases). When lymph node metastases in the neck accompany the tumour a modified cervical node dissection should also be carried out. The risk of permanent hypoparathyroidism and of laryngeal nerve injury is lower than 5% in surgical centres with a large experience in this specialist field. Because of multifocality and local aggressiveness of thyroid cancer in children, surgery should generally be followed by ablation of residual thyroid tissue with I-131. Ablation of thyroid remnants by radioactive iodine is also justified because of their potential interference with further diagnostic procedures. In the follow-up of surgically treated patients unablated residual thyroid tissue may compete with metastatic thyroid lesions for 131-I uptake in the whole body scan and may secrete thyroglobulin preventing its use as a tumour marker. Metastases of differentiated thyroid cancer commonly take up iodine so that diagnostic I-131 can be used in the follow-up of patients to check for distant metastases.

Radioactive iodine can be used to treat lymph node and distant metastases which take up iodine after a total thyroidectomy. In addition, surgical removal of metastatic lesions may also be used when feasible. However, external radiotherapy and/or chemotherapy is usually reserved in the West for the minority of metastases which do not take up radioiodine and cannot be removed surgically.

Thyroid hormone replacement should be carried out with TSH suppressive doses of L-thyroxine, without inducing iatrogenic thyrotoxicosis. For this purpose, concentrations of serum TSH should be kept below 0.1 μU/ml and free triiodothyronine (FT3) concentrations should be maintained within normal limits during treatment.

Optimally treated differentiated childhood thyroid cancer is rarely a fatal disease.

Total or near-total thyroidectomy is only infrequently performed in Belarus, hemi-thyroidectomy or sub-total thyroid resection being the most frequent surgical procedure, in spite of the large proportion of multifocal and locally invasive thyroid cancers. Lymphadenectomy is not routinely performed in patients with cervical lymph node metastases. Most of the surgical procedures are performed in the major referral centre in Minsk, where experienced surgeons are available, although operating theatres and other surgical facilities and equipment are not adequate. Several patients are referred from peripheral centres after primary surgery has been performed elsewhere making management more difficult.

Radioiodine therapy for ablation of thyroid residues and for treatment of functioning metastases is not performed in Belarus because of the virtually total lack of facilities. Consequently external radiotherapy is quite extensively used although this lacks the selectivity of Iodine-131 treatment.

Thyroid hormone medication is performed in Belarus by the administration of different commercial thyroid hormone preparations containing L-triiodothyronine, L-thyroxine or a combination of both. The effectiveness of treatment in suppressing TSH is not routinely assessed by measurement of serum TSH because of lack of resources.

Follow-up

In the West the follow-up of patients is based on clinical examination, ultrasonography of the neck (to detect local recurrence or cervical lymph node metastases) and measurement of serum thyroglobulin (in the absence of any residual normal thyroid, detection of circulating thyroglobulin indicates metastatic disease) (Pacini et al., 1980).

Measurements of serum TSH and thyroid hormones should be performed at regular intervals to monitor the adequacy of thyroid suppressive therapy. Free, rather than total, thyroid hormone concentrations (and, if possible, FT3 rather than FT4) should preferably be determined (Bartalena et al., 1987). Serum anti-thyroglobulin antibody should be measured because of its interference with the measurement of thyroglobulin. Assessment of other antibodies and of other immunological aspects is not diagnostically or therapeutically relevant.

I-131 whole body scanning is performed after withdrawal of thyroxine medication, to assess the efficiency of ablative radioiodine therapy and for the detection of functioning metastases. Chest X-rays are recommended for the detection and follow-up of lung metastases. Bone X-rays and/or scintigraphy are reserved for dubious cases.

In Belarus, the follow-up of children with thyroid cancer is performed mainly in the referral centres of Minsk, but local physicians and peripheral centres are also involved. Thus, standard and common criteria may not easily be applied. Clinical examination, ultrasonography, TSH and thyroid hormone measurements are performed in referral centres at regular intervals, but this may not be the case for other centres. Frequently, measurements of serum thyroglobulin assays are not available at the time of therapeutic decision. Standardisation of the assays used between CIS centres and major European centres would be advantageous.

Iodine-131 whole-body scan for the detection of thyroid remnants and functioning metastases is not performed, because of the lack of appropriate equipment. Chest and bone X-rays are extensively used at fairly frequent intervals.

9. Projection of possible future developments

The Chernobyl accident is the first, and hopefully, the last, reactor accident, with such an enormous release of radioactivity, affecting so many people. Accurate prediction of future thyroid carcinoma development in the exposed population is difficult, because of the lack of any close precedent. There is no doubt that radiation is carcinogenic to the thyroid, both in man and animals (Shore, 1992) but there is no agreement on the relative carcinogenicity of external irradiation (from X-rays) and internal radiation (from isotopes of iodine) (NCRP report No.80). In addition, the dose rate is important but quantitative information on this is lacking.

The perception that radioactive iodine is not carcinogenic in man is largely based on follow-up studies of adults given therapeutic doses of Iodine-131 for Graves' disease or tracer doses for diagnostic purposes (Holm, 1980; 1988). Available data on children submitted to therapeutic or diagnostic procedures with Iodine-131 are scanty and not conclusive. A risk factor derived from the treatment of adult patients with Graves' disease should not be applied to the very different situation of radiation to the thyroid in normal children. Patients with Graves' disease receive radioiodine after the thyroid has undergone a period of growth stimulation, due to the thyroid stimulating antibodies which are the cause of the hyperthyroidism. In normal children exposed to radioiodine from fallout, physiological growth continues after the administration of the isotope, and growth may, if the dose of radiation is large enough, be increased because of post-radiation damage to thyroid function leading to a secondary TSH response. Post-mutagen growth is known to be important in experimental thyroid carcinogenesis and the growth capacity of the thyroid follicular cell is known to be limited (Wynford-Thomas et al, 1982). It is therefore not surprising that radioiodine may be carcinogenic to normal children, but be virtually free of risk (other than hypothyroidism) when used in the treatment of adults for Graves' disease.

A number of studies have been carried out on the occurrence of thyroid carcinoma in irradiated populations and these have very recently been reviewed by R.E. Shore (1992). Two tables from his article have been abstracted and are presented here. The first (Table 9.1) shows the results of 18 estimates of cancer risk from acute external radiation. The range of excess relative risk per Gray for juveniles under the age of 20 is from 2.1 to 36.5, including both cohort and screening studies. For mixed juvenile and adult populations exposed to external radiation the range, of excess relative risk is from zero to 3.30 and for irradiation of adults from zero to 3.1. It is not possible to combine all the studies from the published reports into one overall risk because of the differing balance of ages and number of patients in the different studies, but it is clear that children have a higher relative risk than adults. The studies of thyroid cancer risk from medical exposure to radioactive iodines, atomic weapons fall out or protracted environmental exposure are again based on 18 studies (Table 9.2). The excess relative risk per Gray varies from zero to 3.1 for juvenile exposure, from zero to 0.5 for adult exposure and from zero to 0.3 for adults exposed to high dose Iodine-131 therapy. It again appears that children are more sensitive to the carcinogenic effects of internal irradiation than are adults, but that internal irradiation from I-131 is a less effective carcinogen than external radiation.

TABLE
Estimates of Thyroid Cancer Risk from Acute External Irradiation Before Age 20 or in Adulthood

Study, first author (Reference)	Age at irradiation (y)	No. irradiated persons	Mean year follow-up	Mean dose (Gy)	Observed/expected cancers (90% CI)	Excess RR per Gy (90% CI)	Absolute risk $\times 10^{-4}$ (PY Gy)$^{-1}$
Juvenile irradiation: Cohort studies							
Japanese A-bomb, Akiba (2)	0–9	~8,000	34	0.26	12[b]	5.1 (—)[a]	1.5[c] (—)[a]
	10–19	~8,000	34	0.26	28[b]	2.1 (—)[a]	1.2[c] (—)[a]
Enlarged thymus, Shore (3, 21)	0–1	2,650	36	1.4[d]	37/1.52	8.90 (4.20–21.7)	2.9 (2.1–3.9)
Tinea capitis, Ron (4)	0–15	10,834	30	0.1	43/10.7	27.0 (15.0–42.0)	12.5 (5.8–16)
Tinea capitis, Shore (5)	0–18	2,227	35	0.06	2/1.3	7.70 (0–48.2)	1.5 (0–9.4)
Skin hemangioma, Furst (6, 20)	Mostly <1	14,000	34[c]	0.08	13/7.0	10.12 (1.7–22.2)	2.2 (0.4–4.8)
Childhood cancer therapy, Tucker (7)	0–18	9,100	8	12.5	23/0.43	4.20 (2.90–5.80)	0.4 (0.3–0.6)
Juvenile irradiation: Screening studies							
Lymphoid hyperplasia, Pottern (14)	0–18	1,195	29	0.24	13/2.2[c]	5.86 (1.8–19.1)	15.5 (2.6–58)
Thymus/cervical adenitis, Maxon (13)	Child	1,266	35	2.9	16/2.2[c]	4.50 (2.80–6.90)	1.3 (0.8–2.0)
Tonsil, Schneider (11)[f]	0–14[g]	3,640	35	7.9[d]	242/~4.0[c]	15.20 (13.60–16.90)	3.4 (3.0–3.7)
Tuberculous adenitis, Hanford (84)[f]	<20	38	25	8.2[c]	6/0.02[c]	36.5 (17.4–69)	9.3 (4.4–17)
Tonsil/thymus/acne, De-Groot (62)[f]	Child	263	26	4.5	11/~0.3[c]	12.00 (7.00–19.30)	4.3 (2.5–6.9)
Mixed juvenile and adult irradiation							
Cervical adenitis, Fjalling (17)[f]	0–44	444	43	7.3[c]	25/2.2[c]	3.30 (2.30–4.60)	1.9 (1.4–2.7)
Tuberculous lymphadenitis, van Daal (18)[f]	~16 (Mean)	306	38	10.6	5/0.9	0.5 (0.1–1.0)	0.4 (0.1–0.8)
Hodgkin's therapy,[h] Hancock (85)	2–82	1,677	10	~34[c]	6/0.4	0.4 (0.2–0.8)	0.2 (0.1–0.3)
Tonsil/other, Royce (86)	~19 (Mean)	214	28	7.2[i]	1/1.8	0.0 (0.0–0.3)	0.0 (0.0–1.2)
Adult irradiation							
Japanese A-bomb, Akiba (2)	20–39	~11,000	34	0.26	43[b]	0.8 (—)[a]	0.6[c] (—)[a]
	40+	~11,000	34	0.26	34[b]	0.0 (—)[a]	0.0 (—)[a]
Cervical cancer therapy, Boice (19)	Mostly >30	82,616	8	0.11	43/32[i]	3.1 (0.5–6.5)	2.9 (0.5–6.0)
Tuberculous adenitis, Hanford (84)	20+	124	25 (Screened)	8.2[c]	2/0.2[c]	1.2 (0.2–3.7)	0.9 (0.1–2.6)

Note. The estimates are based on calculations for the interval 5 or more years postirradiation.

[a] Age-specific information was not given.

[b] Includes both irradiated and unirradiated (<0.01 Gy) cases because an age-specific breakdown by dose was not given. Expected values were not given.

[c] Value was estimated for this tabulation based on data presented in the report.

[d] Dosimetry is currently being reevaluated, but new results are not yet available.

[e] Risk estimates were made using an expected value calculated for this tabulation from estimated age-sex specific person-years. For screening studies without an appropriate control group, the estimated general-population expected values were doubled, based on the findings of Prentice *et al.* (12), to help account for screening effects. Estimates of expected values that are especially uncertain are marked with a "~".

[f] These screening studies had no unirradiated group with screening for comparison with the irradiated group.

[g] 297 thyroid cancers were diagnosed, but 55 were reported as "occult sclerosing" type and are not included.

[h] 52% received chemotherapy as well.

[i] Dose to the treated organ; in some cases the thyroid dose may have been much less than that to the treated organ.

[j] Based on their maximum observed and general-population expected. Their original observed number (36 cases) was less and gave lower excess relative risk (ERR) and excess absolute risk (EAR) estimates (ERR = 1.1, 90% CI = −1.4, 4.3; EAR = 1.1, 90% CI = −1.3, 4.0). Their nested case-control study yielded a much higher risk estimate from the dose–response analysis, but with wide confidence intervals because of the small sampling of controls (ERR = 12.3, 90% CI = −5.5, 127; EAR = 6.5, 90% CI = −2.9, 67).

ROY E. SHORE

TABLE

Estimates of Thyroid Cancer Risk from Medical Exposure to Radioactive Iodines, Atomic Weapons Fallout, or Protracted Environmental Exposures

Study, first author (Reference)	Age at irradiation (y)	No. irradiated persons	Mean year Follow-up	Mean dose (Gy)	Observed/expected cancers	Excess RR per Gy (90% CI)	Absolute risk × 10^{-4} (PY Gy) (90% CI)
Juvenile exposure							
Swedish diagnostic ^{131}I, Holm (36)	0–19	~2,000	20	1.6	2/1.2	0.5 (<0–2.6)	0.2 (<0–0.9)
FDA diagnostic ^{131}I, Hamilton (37)	0–20	3,503	27	~0.6[c]	4/1.40	3.1 (<0–2.3)	0.5 (<0–3.5)
Utah ^{131}I fallout, Rallison (87)	0–9	1,962	~32	~0.2[c]	6/9.0	0.0 (0–3.7)	0.0 (0–5.6)
Marshall Islands, Robbins (41, 42)	0–18	127	32	12.4[a]	6/1.2	0.3 (0.1–0.7)	1.1 (0.4–2.3)
Adult exposure							
Swedish diagnostic ^{131}I, Holm (36)	>19	24,200[b]	20	0.42[b]	16/25.8[b]	<0 (<0–<0)	<0 (<0–<0)
German diagnostic ^{131}I, Globel (40)	Adult (mostly)	13,896	~17[c]	1.0[c]	80/63.6	0.3 (0–1.4)[d]	0.9 (0–2.6)[d]
Marshall Islands, Robbins (41, 42)	>18	126	32	4.66[a]	3/0.9	0.5 (0.0–1.6)	1.3 (0.1–3.8)
High-dose ^{131}I therapy							
Swedish hyperthyroidism, Holm (88)	57 (mean)	10,207	15	~113[c]	18/13.3	0.0 (<0–0.0)	0.0 (<0–0.0)
Minnesota hyperthyroidism, Hoffman (89)	57 (mean)	1,005	15	88	3/0.8	0.0 (0.0–0.1)	0.0 (0.0–0.1)
USPHS thyrotoxicosis,[f] Dobyns (90)	48 (median)	19,186	8	88	5/2.4	0.0 (<0–0.1)	0.0 (<0–0.0)
Juvenile hyperthyroidism, combined series (33, 90–97)	0–19	602	~10[c]	~88[c]	2/0.1[c]	0.3 (0.0–0.9)	0.1 (0.0–0.2)

Note. The estimates are based on calculations for the interval 5 or more years postirradiation.

[a] The ^{131}I dose to the Marshall Islanders was only 10–20% of the total dose; the remainder was from short-lived radioiodines and external γ radiation.

[b] Excludes the subgroup that was receiving an ^{131}I examination because of a suspicion of thyroid tumor. It includes a small, but unknown, number of subjects <19 years of age.

[c] Estimated for this tabulation from available data.

[d] Estimated for this tabulation from a dose–response analysis of reported data on exposed persons.

[e] Thyroid dose estimated by extrapolation per MBq from other studies of hyperthyroidism (60).

[f] Includes only those with Graves disease in the USPHS Cooperative Thyrotoxicosis Study.

The excess thyroid cancers reported to have followed radiation have, at the earliest, begun three to five years after irradiation. In most of the series analyzed very few cases were seen before about 10 years post-radiation. Excess numbers of cancers continue to occur for decades, even for as long as 50 years after exposure, although the excess risk may decline after 20 years. Exposure of a large population to high doses of Iodine-131 would therefore be expected to lead to an increase in thyroid carcinoma incidence in exposed children, starting some 5 years after the exposure and continuing for many years.

Estimating and projecting the size of the expected increase, based on the published risk estimates, requires knowledge of the size of the exposed population and the dose received, particularly the dosimetry for children. Accurate information is not available on these points, although 1% of children under 7 years of age in the 30 km zone are said to have received thyroid doses from Iodine-131 in excess of 10 Gray with an additional unknown contribution from short lived isotopes of iodine. The numbers of childhood thyroid cancers so far recorded in Belarus are considerably higher than those found in non-exposed populations, and past studies point to the likelihood that the rates will continue to increase for the foreseeable future.

Several aspects of the reported incidence of childhood thyroid cancer in Belarus and the Ukraine are worthy of comment. The latent period is short, but not without precedent. The type of thyroid tumour is largely papillary carcinoma, as has been reported in previous studies of radiation induced tumours. A majority of the tumours show direct extrathyroid invasion and lymph node spread, an unusually high frequency compared with most studies of papillary thyroid cancer in adults, but in keeping with the findings in thyroid cancer in young children (Schlumberger et al, 1987). Both follicular and papillary carcinoma may be associated with previous irradiation and follicular adenomas have also been reported to be increased. No increase of the number of adenomas has been reported in Belarus but as benign lesions are largely dealt with in clinics in the towns in which they present and the published statistics on the malignant tumours are derived from the experience in the Minsk centre, to which selected patients with proven or suspected thyroid carcinoma are referred, it is not possible to provide accurate information at present. It should be remembered that papillary carcinoma appears to derive directly from follicular cells while follicular carcinoma is in many cases thought to be a malignant progression of a pre-existing follicular adenoma. The development of papillary carcinomas post-radiation may not necessarily follow the same time course as the development of the follicular adenoma/carcinoma sequence.

In summary, current data do not allow an accurate prediction of the future extent of the thyroid cancer problem in Belarus and the Ukraine but, based on the estimated dosimetry and previous experience, an increased rate of thyroid carcinoma would be expected in those exposed as children, and an excess of cases of thyroid cases would be expected to continue for decades. The present reported excess of thyroid carcinoma in children is considerable and both this and the dosimetry suggest that it is likely that there will be a sizeable and long continued increase in thyroid carcinoma incidence. **The number of childhood thyroid cancers reported in Belarus together with the Ukraine is approaching the total number of all types of cancers which have been ascribed over the past 40 years to Atomic Bomb Explosions in Japan.** In the population of Rongelap in the Marshall Islands, exposed to fallout from a nuclear test, as well as an increase in cases of thyroid cancer, cases of hypothyroidism have been noted (Dobbyns, 1992). The occurrence of this problem in the future as an occasional long-term consequence of exposure to fallout from Chernobyl can not be discounted. Because there is likely to be a long-term continued considerable increase in thyroid carcinoma incidence, it is most important that steps be taken now to provide help for the care of the current and future patients.

It is crucial that the consequences of this major accident are very carefully monitored and the reasons which lie behind this unanticipated increase in childhood thyroid cancers be thoroughly understood both from a mechanistic and epidemiological point of view so that the European Community and the world as a whole can make rational and informed decisions on radiological protection in the future.

10.   Current international actions

It would be incorrect to complete this report without trying to give some impression of the many International and bilateral efforts of medical help being provided for the people affected by the Chernobyl accident. In the first place the authorities in Belarus, the Ukraine and the Russian Federation have mounted a tremendous effort to monitor the health of the exposed populations and to provide, within the limited means at their disposal, as good a treatment as possible of the health effects arising in that population. In addition, several international agencies including the World Health Organisation (WHO), UNESCO, the International Atomic Energy Agency (IAEA), the Food and Agriculture Organisation (FAO), the International Red Cross, the Council of Europe, the Commission of the European Communities, are all involved in projects to provide help to the affected populations in the three republics. And last, but by no means least, there are many bilateral activities between the three republics and individual nations or charitable foundations, including Japan, and the Sasakawa Foundation, USA, France, Germany, the Netherlands, Finland. Indeed, there are so many different initiatives that it is impossible at present to get a complete coordinated overview of all of the activities so that the following paragraphs should only be seen as an incomplete report on those activities which are in some way concerned with the thyroid consequences of the Chernobyl accident.

The Panel is grateful to the individuals who contributed to the individual sections in this Chapter, WHO, Dr. Ryabukin, WHO Europe, Dr. Baverstock, USA, Dr. Wachholz, Japan, Professor Nagataki, Germany, Professor Reiners, France Dr. Fragu, Switzerland, Professor Egloff and the Netherlands, Dr. Wagemaker.

10.1.   WHO / IPHECA

The **thyroid** project aims at detection and characterization of selected thyroid diseases in children living in the strictly controlled zones (areas where levels of contamination with radiocaesium are higher than 15 Ci/km^2, i.e. 550 kBq/m^2). The diseases of concern are thyroid cancer, benign tumours, autoimmune thyroiditis and hypothyroidism, as it is known that these diseases can be caused by exposure to radiation. The total number of children to be included in the investigation may reach 75 000 in all three States.

To allow comparisons, clinical and epidemiological investigations should be carried out according to a standardized protocol common to all three affected States. A draft protocol was prepared in May 1992 by specialists of the three States in cooperation with WHO. It was then reviewed in July 1992 by an international group of experts. Their recommendations were taken into account in the finalisation of the protocol by experts from the three States in late 1992. In finalising the protocol, constraints on implementing it on the basis of the existing infrastructure had to be reconciled with demands for strict full-scale epidemiological studies on the one hand and the limited resources and time available for carrying out the pilot project on the other.

A very important task within the pilot project is the strengthening of local capability for the early detection of thyroid cancer. To this end 16 ultrasonic instruments were provided through WHO, which can be used both for thorough examinations of the thyroid in hospitals and for field missions. Another contribution was the procurement of instruments and kits for radioimmunoassay and enzyme immunoassay to determine thyroid function and to monitor the treatment of thyroid cancer. Up to 100 national staff have received in country training in the use of the new instrumentation, and scientists have been sponsored to study abroad. Agreements have been reached with institutions in other countries to train a number of specialists both in using instrumentation and in mastering specific techniques (ultrasonography, hormone analysis, morphology, and reconstruction of doses from radioiodine).

10.2 WHO Europe

The European Regional Office of the WHO has prepared an integrated research and technical assistance project based on a network of proposed WHO Collaborating Centres to undertake collaborative work with a proposed WHO Collaborating Centre to be instituted in Minsk. The primary aims of the project will be to create a framework in which research and training aimed at improving diagnosis and treatment of the disease, and investigating the origin, nature and likely extent of the outbreak of thyroid cancer can be conducted in a coherent way in collaboration with Belarussian physicians and scientists.

The Initially proposed Collaborating Centres outside Belarus are the Department of Endocrinology, University of Pisa, Italy; the Department of Histopathology, University of Cambridge, United Kingdom; the Department of Public Health, University of Berne, Switzerland; the Department of Endocrinology, University of Nagasaki, Japan; the Department of Radiobiology, University of Munich, Germany; and the Department of Nuclear Medicine, Institute Gustave-Roussy, Villejuif, France.

These are centres of excellence in the following disciplines: treatment of thyroid cancer, aetiological diagnosis and pathogenesis of thyroid cancer, public health epidemiology, clinical diagnosis of thyroid cancer, dosimetry of iodine isotopes and nuclear medicine. They all have international reputations for their expertise and are integrated into the international community relevant to their particular disciplines. They are all located in countries with a strong interest in the health consequences of exposure to ionising radiations and are well integrated into national research programmes in this area. They are thus well placed to become centres for research activity and will provide links for Belarussian physicians and scientists with the wider international scientific community. All the centres have wide European links, and will be encouraged to involve a wide range of other institutes in cooperative projects.

The project has been approved in Belarus and efforts to attract funding are under way. In anticipation of the project a number of initiatives have been taken including arranging the visit of two physicians to Pisa for training in endocrinology, the visit of one pathologist to Cambridge for research and training and the visit of one scientist to Nagasaki to participate in a survey of the intensity screening activities by region in Belarus.

10.3. USA

Joint Cooperation between the United States and Belarus, Russia and the Ukraine on studies of health effects associated with the Chernobyl nuclear power plant accident

The Union of Soviet Socialist Republics and the United States entered into an agreement in 1988 to carry out joint studies relating to civilian nuclear reactor safety, including environmental and health studies; these joint studies were to be under the direction of a Joint Coordinating Committee for Civilian Nuclear Reactor Safety (JCCCNRS). In March, 1993 this agreement was renewed with Russia, the Ukraine and the United States participation. A separate continuing agreement between Belarus and the United States for environmental and health studies was signed in April 1992. The responsible JCCCNRS coordinators for health-related studies are the U.S. Department of Energy, the Ministers of Health of Belarus and Ukraine, and the Russian Academy of Medical Sciences. The U.S. Department of Energy invited the U.S. National Cancer Institute to be the primary U.S. participant in studies related to cancer.

A number of joint studies to investigate health effects, primarily thyroid disease, particularly cancer, in children and leukaemia in cleanup workers, that may be associated with exposure to radiation as a consequence of the Chernobyl nuclear power plant accident have been or are being developed and/or implemented.

These joint studies are primarily epidemiological in design and contain major components including radiation dosimetry and dose reconstruction, clinical and medical follow up, laboratory analyses, histopathology as appropriate, data acquisition, management and analyses, consultative and administrative procedures, and communication technologies. There are provisions also for training, logistical support, equipment and supplies, etc.

In Belarus, a case-control study of 119 cases of thyroid cancer in children was initiated in 1992 (although at present the reported number of cases is substantially greater). Control subjects for these cases have been selected, the histopathology of the cases has been reviewed by European and American pathologists, and the reconstruction of the radiation dose to the thyroid of each case and control subject has begun. This study is expected to be completed in 1994.

A cohort of at least 15,000 children has been identified for a long-term health follow up epidemiology study for thyroid disease, particularly thyroid cancer. The scientific research protocol for this study recently was completed and has been submitted to the relevant authorities in both countries for their review and consideration. This study is expected to continue for at least 15-20 years, in addition to the participation of appropriate medical and scientific personnel in the Ministry of Health of Belarus, experts from the Institute of Biophysics in Moscow also are participating in these studies with American physicians and scientists.

In the Ukraine joint efforts have been made to develop three cooperative studies: First, case-control study of children with thyroid cancer has been defined and is now being initiated, including the identification of control subjects, histopathology, and the reconstruction of individual thyroid doses. Second, the scientific research protocol for a long-term health follow up epidemiology study for thyroid disease, particularly cancer, is close to completion and is expected to be submitted to both governments for review later this year. The cohort of study subject is expected to include a minimum of 50,000 children. Third, a study protocol that will address the follow up of cleanup workers, particularly with respect to haematological diseases, has been jointly prepared by the Ukrainian and the American physicians and scientists and also is expected to be completed later this year for submission to both governments for review. These joint studies will involve both Ukrainian and American physicians and scientists and the follow up studies are expected to continue for at least 15-20 years.

Discussions are in progress in Russia with respect to the development of a joint study focusing on thyroid disease, particularly cancer, among children exposed to radiation at the time of and following the Chernobyl accident. This study would be similar to those identified in the above paragraphs in Belarus and the Ukraine. Joint studies of haematological disorders among the cleanup workers also are under discussion.

Representatives of the United States and the Commission of the European Communities have made efforts to coordinate their respective studies in order to maximize their productivity and minimize overlap.

10.4. Japan

The "Joint Japan-USSR Seminars on Radiological Medicine" were held in June 1990 and January 1991 in Tokyo to discuss the health consequences of the Chernobyl accident. A cooperative dosimeter study of internal radiation exposure was thus initiated between the both countries.

In April 1991, an agreement on cooperation in mitigation of the health consequences among residents of the affected areas due to the Chernobyl accident was formally signed by the Japanese Prime Minister and Soviet President. It was agreed that cooperation would be extended in studies involving the following four areas: (1) Estimation of radiation doses in whole body and thyroid; (2) Thyroid disorders; (3) Leukaemia and preleukemic conditions; (4) Data management of the exposed individuals.

Protocols dealing with these four projects were prepared and exchange of scientists on these topics is now under way. During these periods, in September 1990, Japanese specialists were engaged in the IAEA (International Atomic Energy Agency) projects.

The Japanese Government provided approximately 20 million US dollars to WHO in February 1991 for the purpose of making available medical equipment and supplies through the WHO ICRHI (International Centre on Radiation Health Issues) which is to be established in Obninsk.

Although many groups and organisations in Japan have extended cooperation in various forms in relation to the Chernobyl accident, notable are the following projects:

<u>Chernobyl Sasakawa Medical and Health Cooperation Project</u> At the beginning of 1990, the Soviet Union made a request to the Sasakawa Foundation for assistance that would

directly help the exposed residents since most of the international and binational agreements related to the Chernobyl accident primarily involved studies and research.

The Foundation decided to provide 40 million US dollars over a five-year period beginning from 1991 in order to conduct the following kinds of cooperation at the five centres in the Republics of Ukraine, Belarus and Russia: (1) Donation of five mobile examination units (with ultrasound equipment for the examination of thyroid, haemoanalysis equipment, whole body counter, etc.) and five buses; (2) Provision of medical equipment and supplies; (3) Provision of medical drugs and reagents; (4) Sending of experts; (5) Acceptance of trainees; (6) Educational activities for the residents of the affected areas.

These projects are going on smoothly with emphasis on the following three points and priority on children: (1) Haematological disturbances; (2) Thyroid disorders; (3) Radiation dosimetry.

The Hiroshima International Council for Medical Care of the Radiation Exposed (HICARE) Although cooperation in the area of medical care for the Chernobyl accident had been extended previously by various radiation-related institutions in Hiroshima, this Council was organised in 1991 to conduct such cooperation more effectively. The activities to be carried out are as follows: (1) Acceptance of physicians for training and sending of experts; (2) Preparation of reference documents on medical care for exposed people; (3) Education and dissemination of information.

Active work was begun in all of these three areas from April 1991 with an annual budget of about 540,000 US dollars.

Nagasaki Association for Hibakushas' Medical Care This association has been established since April 1922, for the purpose of giving out aid and practical information for radiation victims and to invite leading medical specialists actively involved in helping the victims from the Chernobyl accident. Annual budget is about 270,000 US dollars.

10.5. Project of the German Joint Committee on Radiation Research :
"Scientists Aid Children of Chernobyl"

In 1990, seven scientific organisations formed the Joint Committee for Radiation Research. The main focus of this committee is the coordination of radiation research projects and the representation of the German Associations in the IAAR: Society for Biophysics; German Society for Medical Physics; German Society for Nuclear Medicine; German Society of Physics; German Roentgen Society; Association for Radiation Protection; and Association of German Physicians in Radiation Protection.

In 1991, the Joint Committee decided to plan a project primarily designed to give humanitarian help to children who developed thyroid cancer in Belarus after the reactor accident of Chernobyl. The Committee succeeded in gaining a grant of approximately 3 Million Deutsch Mark from German Industrial Companies for this subject.

On February 23rd and 24th 1993, the Minister of Health of Belarus, His Excellency V. Kazakov, Professor E. Demidchik, Director of Thyroid Tumour Centre of Belarus and Professor L. Asthakova, Deputy Director of State Institute for Radiation Medicine visited Essen, Germany, to establish and sign the protocol for this project.

The protocol has three sub-projects: 1) Optimisation of treatment of thyroid cancer in children living in the contaminated areas of Belarus led by Professor Ch. Reiners, University of Essen; 2) Evaluation of biological indicators of early detection and optimisation of therapy led by Prof. C. Streffer, University of Essen; 3) Dosimetry and risk analysis led by Dr H. Paretzke, Institute for Radiation Protection, Neuherberg).

Because humanitarian help and optimisation of treatment is the main focus of the protocol, the project is organised centrally by Professor Ch. Reiners. In this context, the following support will be offered to the Belarussian partners in the project who are represented by Professor E. Demidchik:

1)   Advice to Belarussian physicians in surgery, nuclear medicine radiation therapy, endocrinology and paediatrics by German specialists with respect to treatment of thyroid cancer;

2)   Provision of surgical instruments, material and drugs urgently needed for treatment of thyroid cancer in children;

3)   Training of Belarussian physicians in surgery, nuclear medicine, radiation therapy, endocrinology and paediatrics in Germany with respect to treatment of thyroid cancer;

4)   Selection and transfer of Belarussian children with thyroid cancer for special

treatment in Germany (i.e. I-131 therapy) as long as this treatment is not available

in Belarus;

5)   Consultation to plan and establish facilities for I-131 therapy for thyroid cancer in

Belarus by German specialists.

Exchange of physicians and transfer of patients will be organised by coordination centres

in Essen (D) and Minsk (Belarus). The project starts on April 1993.

10.6. The Netherlands-Belarussian humanitarian aid project

The principal participant, the Dutch Ministry of Welfare, Health and Cultural Affairs

established a project running from 1 September 1991 to 31 August 1993 with the Ministry

of Health of Belarus. The Dutch Ministry is represented by the Bureau for International

Cooperation of the National Institute for Public Health and Environmental Protection,

and the University Hospital of Utrecht and the aim of the project is to provide

humanitarian assistance to people with complaints which are attributed to the Chernobyl

Nuclear Power Plant Disaster.

On March 8, 1991, the Dutch Council of Ministers approved the Gomel project and

made an amount of 10 Million Dutch guilders (4.5 MioECU) available for a project

period of two years starting on September 1, 1991, to provide humanitarian assistance

to people with complaints which are attributed to the Chernobyl Nuclear Power Plant

disaster. The Dutch Ministry of Welfare, Health and Cultural Affairs charged the

National Institute of Public Health and Environmental Protection (RIVM) with the responsibility for the execution of the project. The counterpart of the RIVM for project execution is the Belarussian Ministry of Health and the University Hospital of Utrecht is a partner in the project. The Project activities are centred on the Gomel Regional Specialized Polyclinic, the Gomel Health Information Centre and a polyclinic and a hospital in Minsk. The project involves the provision of technical assistance and training of Belarussian medical staff and includes the purchase of (medical) equipment, (medical) furniture, audiovisual equipment, reagents and medicine. Preparatory activities took place during the period of June 1 - August 31, 1991, and the Project commenced on September 1, 1991, for a duration of two years.

The project consists of three phases:

Phase I (duration 6 months) concerned the training of Belarussian staff at the University Hospital in Utrecht. Two Dutch medical specialists and a nurse were stationed in Gomel to provide technical assistance to the Belarussian medical staff and nurses. During Phase I, further areas were identified where additional expert advice and training activities were needed and this specialised additional training was provided on a regular basis by means of short-term missions of expert staff to Gomel. The first batches of equipment were procured during this Phase and the Gomel Polyclinic started functioning on November 18, 1991. Dr. Kazakov, Belarussian Minister of Health and Dr. Garvalink, Chairman of the Project Steering Committee (replacing the Ambassador to the Netherlands), officially opened the Gomel Polyclinic on January 30, 1992.

Phase II (duration 15 months) is concerned with a continuation of the activities initiated and defined in detail during Phase I. Medical specialists provide technical assistance in Gomel and Belarussian staff are trained in Gomel and in The Netherlands. Additional equipment has been procured during Phase II. A plan of activities for dealing with psycho-social problems was formulated and is presently being carried out, the training activities having started in June 1992. A plan to set up an information campaign for the population living in the affected areas of Belarus has also been prepared and training activities for this component of the Project started in August 1992. A Belarussian-Dutch Health Information Centre was opened to the general public in Gomel in mid-September 1992. Some activities which will be at the national level (in Minsk)and will focus on post-graduate training, initially concentrating on endocrinology, have also been defined and are planned to be implemented as of January 1993. Medical and laboratory equipment, audio-visual equipment, reagents, etc., were supplied to Hospital 10 and the Republican Endocrinological Dispensary in Minsk during the last week of November 1992 and a Dutch Medical Specialist has been stationed in Minsk from January 1993.

Phase III (duration 3 months) will be the "handing-over" Phase. During this period, the role of the Dutch staff will be limited to an advisory one so that the Belarussian staff will carry out all of the activities dealt with during the previous Phases.

10.7. Swiss Activities in Support of Belarus

Fund for the Support of Eastern European Countries: The Swiss Federal Office of Foreign Economy has proposed that 600 Mio Swiss Francs be made available to support activities in the former Soviet Union, although this has yet to be approved by the National Council in the spring session. 10 Mio SFr. of this fund would be used for activities on health and environment problems, but there are no plans at present which specifically target Belarus.

Funds for Research into Health Effects after Chernobyl: The Swiss Federal Health Office has proposed that 1 Mio SFr./year for 1993, 1994 and 1995 should be invested in cooperation with the Rome office of WHO Europe, although this may be reduced because of a lack of Federal finances. There will be a convention in Berne on January 29, 1993 to discuss how this money will be spent.

Doctors for the Environment, Group "Chernobyl": To date some 200,000 SFr. have been invested in providing drugs, infusions, X-ray equipment,etc to the hospital at Lesnoj as well as supporting the exchange of doctors. The Woloshin Programme is especially concerned with a dental caries prophylaxis programme. In addition there is a Red Cross Programme in Mogilev which works through outpatient treatment providing primary medical needs and pharmaceuticals.

Electricity Companies of the Canton of Berne : A computer has been provided for the cancer registry of Belarus in Lesnoj, Minsk.

Doctors for Social Responsibility and Swiss Paediatric Oncology group: A programme for the exchange of doctors, nurses and laboratory technicians has been established with the help of "Glückskette".

10.8. Project "Franco-Ukranian Centre"

A Franco-Ukranian Centre was set up in Kiev, Ukraine, in 1991. The French participants are C. Parmentier and M. Schlumberger, Institut Gustave-Roussy; J.C. Nenot, N. Parmentier, Institut de Sureté et de Protection Nucléaire; and the Association "Les Enfants de Chernobyl" ("Children of Chernobyl"), under the auspices of the Ministry of Health and the Humanitarian Aid.

The aim of this centre was to assess the thyroid and the haematological status of the children who were in Pripyat (within the 10 km zone of the reactor) at the time of the accident and were then evacuated to Kiev. The targeted population was about 7000 children, and in a second stage their families (20 000 adults). The centre is equipped with ultrasound machines, and with blood cell counters. Three million FF were allocated to equip the centre and half a million are donated annually for maintenance of the project. The French participation was planned for two years and now the centre is run by the Ukranians.

11. Recommendations - Actions

11.A. Technical assistance

Thyroid cancer in children does not have to be a lethal disease if it is treated optimally as soon as it is diagnosed. The Ministry of Health and the surgeons and doctors in Belarus are doing remarkable work but they are badly handicapped because there is a severe shortage of modern therapeutic equipment and, consequently, little training in the most up-to-date treatment procedures. This is a serious situation, and one in which the European Community could take and play a pivotal role by providing the essential Technical Assistance as a complete package.

A.1 Aims

Technical assistance is needed to improve the infrastructure of medical services in the republics of Belarus, Russia and the Ukraine with respect to diagnosis, therapy and follow-up of thyroid cancer in children. Programmes for technical assistance must be realized step by step, starting with the training of physicians, nurses and technicians. Specialists in surgery, nuclear medicine, pathology, radiotherapy, endocrinology and paediatrics should be involved. After initial training, a complete package of technical equipment has to be supplied. The last step of a technical assistance programme must be continuing support concerning training and supply of materials which could be realized in the context of rotating fellowships.

The final aim of such a program will be multilateral cooperation on medical diagnosis, therapy and follow-up of thyroid cancer in children as well as on research projects concerning radiation induction of such cancers.

A.2. Realisation

The first step will be the bilateral formulation of projects by centres of the CIS countries and the CEC. The projects have to be realized as partnerships between Eastern and Western hospitals and research institutions. With the financial support of the CEC, medical staff (physicians, nurses, technicians) will be invited to visit hospitals in the EC specializing in the diagnosis, treatment and follow-up of thyroid cancer. In the same way, research personnel will visit relevant research institutions in European Community countries.

The programme should enable senior physicians and scientists of CIS countries to become familiar with the special methods used for diagnosis, therapy and follow-up of thyroid cancer as well as with methods used in radiation dosimetry and biology. This will usually be achieved by relatively short visits to EC centres (2 - 4 weeks). Staff personnel (fellows, nurses, technicians) should then have the possibility of staying for longer periods (several months) at Western institutions. After gaining experience in the methods which they will later establish in their home countries, they will be asked to apply for the equipment and material required for such projects. This application will be assisted by the EC partner centre. After delivery of equipment and material financed by the CEC, medical and research partners of Community countries will support CIS partners concerning implementation of technical procedures, quality control and continuing education.

A.3 Diagnosis of thyroid cancer in children

Ultrasonography is the method of choice for early detection of thyroid nodules. The WHO IPHECA programme and the Sasakawa Foundation of Japan have provided Belarus, Russia and the Ukraine with modern ultrasound equipment, so it would not seem to be necessary to provide additional support concerning this type of equipment. However, training and assistance in the quality control of sonography of the thyroid has to be recommended.

Sonography does not permit benign tumours to be differentiated from the malignant thyroidal lesions. The only investigation sufficiently accurate to confirm the diagnosis of papillary carcinoma preoperatively is cytology after fine needle aspiration biopsy. Support for equipment (eg. microtomes and microscopes) and material (glass slides, etc.) is necessary, as well as training and assistance in quality control.

Facilities for the processing, sectioning and staining of the resected thyroid tissue are also limited, and modern equipment (e.g. microtomes) and consumables are both required. There is little or no experience in the use of immunohistochemistry in tumour diagnosis and materials for these investigations or cooperation with a European centre to carry out the studies is needed. In addition technical training in the use of modern techniques is recommended.

A.4   Treatment of thyroid cancer in children

The prerequisites for thyroid surgery in children in several centres in Belarus are far from optimal. This includes much of the facilities needed for anaesthesia, surgery and hospital hygiene; for example, instruments for surgery in children and suture materials are lacking. Assistance is needed to enable anaesthetists and surgeons to increase their expertise in the particular anaesthetic and surgical procedures required for the optimal care of thyroid cancer in children and to provide them with the equipment and materials required.

Facilities for radioiodine treatment of thyroid cancer, equipped with scanner, gamma cameras, etc., are almost completely lacking in these centres in Belarus which are concerned in the treatment of thyroid cancer in children. Assistance is required to provide this equipment and relevant materials (radionuclides, films, etc.). Specialist, training will be needed for those handling the radioiodine, the operation and quality control of equipment, radiation protection and medical applications.

Radical surgery of the thyroid, may be complicated by hypoparathyroidism and paresis of the laryngeal nerve. Training of specialists in Western centres will help to reduce the frequency of such complications to a very low level and to provide appropriate treatment where such complications unavoidably occur.

All the children adequately treated will be hypothyroid and must receive replacement therapy with L-thyroxine in TSH-suppressive doses for the rest of their lives. Centres should be provided with drugs of sufficient quality necessary for medical treatment.

A.5   Follow-up of thyroid cancer in children

Laboratory procedures for the determination of serum TSH, thyroid hormones (T3 and T4) or preferable free thyroid hormones (FT3 and FT4), thyroglobulin and anti-thyroglobulin antibody are of the utmost importance for the follow-up of patients with thyroid cancer. Arrangements must be made for high quality reagent kits from selected manufacturers to be supplied on a long-term basis. The performance of these kits must be tested under local conditions before clinical application. Laboratory personnel must be well trained because, during clinical use of the kits, quality control at a high level is mandatory. Centres for treatment and follow-up of thyroid cancer in children must be equipped with scanners or, preferably, gamma cameras for radioiodine scans to check for metastases.

A.6.   Iodine deficiency

The fraction of ingested radioiodide taken up by the thyroid of a normal individual, and therefore, the dose to this organ, is inversely related to the dietary iodine supply of this individual. In countries where this supply is high (e.g., the USA) the uptake is around 15 to 20%; in countries with mild iodine deficiency (e.g., Belgium) it is around 45 to 60%. Increasing iodine supply in a country could therefore reduce the radiation load after a nuclear accident by a fraction of three, but unfortunately iodide dietary supplementation was discontinued in Southern Belarus shortly before the nuclear accident.

Experimental work has shown that the optimal protocol for inducing thyroid tumours in animals is the administration of radioiodide followed by thyroid stimulation by iodine deficiency or thyroid blockade. Tumorigenesis depends on the duration and extent of thyroid stimulation. Conversely, after thyroid irradiation, treatments which decrease thyroid stimulation reduce tumorigenesis.

Treatments available for such a purpose would be iodine dietary supplementation, or L-thyroxine oral administration. To be effective thyroxine treatment would involve medical treatment of a whole population, or defined fraction of this population. It would be very costly and difficult to control and might involve iatrogenic disease from excessive dosage. Iodine supplementation would decrease the level of thyroid stimulation in the whole population by indirect inhibition of thyrotropin secretion from the resulting higher levels of thyroxine. To be effective, such supplementation should raise daily dietary intake to at least 150 μg/day. This could be achieved by supplying iodide tablets to the population or by salt iodination. The latter solution, which can be applied indefinitely and does not require extensive distribution services, is preferable.

A side benefit of iodine prophylaxis would be to decrease markedly the incidence of goitre in the population. Also by reducing this incidence and thus the general frequency of nodular goitres it would decrease the background of nodularity which may mask the appearance of radiation induced thyroid cancers.

11.B.   Research Cooperation in the development of skills

Diagnosis and treatment of thyroid carcinomas, as well as work involved in understanding the pathology of thyroid carcinoma, require the involvement of a range of specialists. The study of radiation-induced hypothyroidism and its relationship with thyroid autoimmunity and thyroid tumorigenesis also requires a multidisciplinary approach. To improve co-operation between the CIS and the CEC, it is suggested that a series of research projects be created, for example under the current CHECIR APAS programme to allow scientists from the CIS involved in the diagnosis and treatment of patients with thyroid carcinoma, or in research related to radiation and thyroid carcinoma, to work together with scientists from comparable recognised centres in the EC. If possible the project should allow for the extended visit of scientists from the CIS to the centres in the EC so that a research project could be undertaken during the visit, with the possibility of further co-operation in the future, leading to the forging of links between centres in the CIS and centres in the EC.

B.1   Development of protocols for prevention and management of disease

It is proposed that a research project be established to define a set of protocols aimed at the rationalisation and optimalisation of the treatment of childhood thyroid cancer.

As pointed out in the previous section, current prevention and management procedures used in Belarus are not always consistent with the standards of practice in the West and need to be adjusted, taking into account the local conditions which influence diagnostic, therapeutic and follow-up measures. This justifies the need for the development of specific protocols to be devised in collaboration with the Belarus medical and surgical centres and also with comparable centres in the Ukraine and the Russian Federation. Such protocols should consider screening methods; clinical laboratory and instrumental diagnostic procedures; handling of the resected tissue; surgical and post-surgical therapeutic measures; follow-up schedules and other related aspects.

Protocols should also be developed for thyroid disorders other than thyroid carcinoma. These include hypothyroidism, which may result from thyroid irradiation; benign thyroid nodules, which may also be induced by thyroid irradiation as well as nontoxic goitre, both nodular and non-nodular, which is more prevalent in areas of iodine deficiency such as Belarus.

B.2. The Molecular, Cellular and Biological Characterisation of Childhood Thyroid Tumours

Malignancy results from interaction between the genetic make-up of the individual and the environment. In the aftermath of Chernobyl this interaction took place on an unprecedented scale. Research into the thyroid effects of the exposure of millions of people to fallout from Chernobyl is vitally important to provide complete or partial answers to a number of questions. These include :

1.	How sensitive are humans to the carcinogenic effect of exposure to isotopes of iodine ? Can this effect be quantified as an excess relative risk per Gray ?

2.   Are children more sensitive than adults and can this relative sensitivity be
      quantified ?

3.   What is the importance of short lived isotopes of iodine in the link between
      radiation exposure and thyroid carcinoma ?

4.   Are the cancers induced by exposure to radioactive contamination morphologically
      different from spontaneous cancers ? Do all the major types of thyroid cancer
      occur following exposure to radiation from radioactive contamination ?

5.   What oncogenes and tumour suppressor genes are important in thyroid
      carcinogenesis. Is the pattern of oncogene activation found in thyroid cancers
      induced by internal or external radiation different from that seen in spontaneous
      thyroid carcinomas ? If so, can these observations be used to help to determine
      the likelihood that thyroid cancer in any one individual is due to radiation ?

6.   Is the clinical behaviour of thyroid carcinomas induced by exposure to internal or
      external radiation different from that spontaneous thyroid carcinoma in the same
      age groups ? If so, are different therapeutic approaches required ? Can any
      differing clinical behaviour be correlated with the morphological or molecular
      biological changes in the tumour concerned ?

7.	What environmental factors contributed to the exposure of individuals who later developed thyroid carcinoma ? What factors after the initial exposure to radiation affected the likelihood of progression to malignancy ?

8.	Is the time of onset of radiation induced thyroid carcinoma related to the dose of radiation and to the age at radiation ?

9.	Does radiation from radioactive iodine increase the risk of benign as well as malignant thyroid tumours ? Is there evidence of progression from benign to malignant tumours both in radiation and non-radiation induced thyroid malignancy ?

10.	To what extent are changes in thyroid autoimmunity relevant to the effects of radiation on the thyroid ?

11.	What is the relevance of radiation-induced hypothyroidism in relation to thyroid tumorigenesis and thyroid autoimmunity ?

To attempt to provide answers to these and to other relevant questions will require molecular biological, histopathological and experimental work linked to epidemiological and clinical studies.

Clinical Studies

To provide information on which future work may be based it is necessary to ensure that there is careful and consistent investigation and documentation for each case of thyroid carcinoma. A standard set of investigations should be carried out on each patient, including for example thyroid function tests and thyroid antibody measurements. These should be carried out by sensitive reproducible techniques and methodology regularly checked by external quality control. A standard protocol should be drawn up to be completed for each patient. This should list not only the clinical details and operative findings but also questions relevant to an assessment of exposure to radioactive contamination from Chernobyl. Appropriate investigations on family members should also be undertaken.

Histopathology

The nature of the diagnosis of each new case must be established reliably with modern techniques and with consistent protocols. The resected tissue should be carefully treated and some tumour tissue frozen on resection and stored at -70°. Other tissue must be fixed and processed in a way which will allow accurate diagnosis and will preserve DNA in a state which will allow the use of Polymerase Chain reaction (PCR) and other molecular biological techniques in the future. Extensive sampling of tissue, both tumour and background thyroid should be undertaken to ensure that there is an adequate supply of research materials for future study. Whenever possible a blood sample separated into cell and plasma fractions should also be stored.

The histopathological features in these thyroid carcinomas in children should be carefully compared with those in childhood thyroid cancer unrelated to radiation. Changes in the type of thyroid cancer observed with age of the patient should be studied as should changes in the background presumed irradiated but non-neoplastic thyroid. It is important that material from thyroidectomies carried out in the peripheral clinics as well as from the centre should also be collected to allow study of the incidence and histological type of benign tumours and to confirm the validity of diagnoses made in the peripheral clinics.

Molecular Biology

The nature of the oncogene and tumour suppressor gene changes occurring in thyroid cancer should be better defined and correlated with the histological type of thyroid cancer and the age of the patient. A specific study of oncogene changes in the radiation-induced and non-radiation-induced series of thyroid carcinomas should be undertaken, including the oncogenes *ret* and *trk* known to be activated by gene rearrangement in a minority of unselected papillary carcinomas. These rearrangements could well be induced by radiation more frequently than, for example, point mutations in the *ras* genes. Techniques to apply these studies to paraffin embedded tissues (e.g. in situ hybridisation) should be developed to allow study of archival material. Investigations of oncogene changes in radiation induced experimental thyroid carcinomas in animals would provide useful information on tumours where there is no doubt that radiation was the carcinogenetic agent.

Experimental Work

The ability of Iodine-131 to induce thyroid tumours in experimental animals is well documented but, there is no good evidence on the comparative oncogenicity of the short lived isotopes of Iodine and Iodine-131. Experimental studies of the consequences of exposure to different doses of Iodine-132 and Iodine-131 with and without subsequent elevation of TSH (using chronic goitrogen treatment) should be undertaken. In addition, further studies could be undertaken of the relation between growth and the susceptibility to mutagenesis and oncogenesis in the thyroid to aid in understanding the apparent discrepancy between the lack of oncogenicity of Iodine-131 when used in the treatment of thyrotoxicosis and when ingested by children from radioactive contamination.

Epidemiology

Epidemiology studies must include case control studies to illuminate the relationship between the development of thyroid malignancy and the many factors that might be relevant to the causation of the malignancy. These include the estimated total thyroid dose and the estimated dose from the different isotopes. Because, however, of the uncertainty attached to these estimations the primary data should also be compared to the age, sex, location at the time of the Chernobyl accident and living habits, for example sleeping outside, and eating habits, for example milk intake, especially milk from "private cows". Longterm follow-up studies of a cross-section of the population exposed to radioactive contamination from Chernobyl are obviously necessary. These should be planned to last for at least 20 years. Appropriate family studies should be undertaken.

Joint epidemiological, pathological and clinical studies should be undertaken urgently to relate the incidence of thyroid carcinoma to exposure from radioactive contamination from Chernobyl by studying that informative group of children born just before or within 6 months of the event and those born in the succeeding few years. Providing screening is continued at the existing level of intensity through this critical period, it should be possible within a short time to establish whether or not there is a dramatic drop in the incidence of thyroid cancer in children born more than 6 months after the Chernobyl disaster. This will provide one of the most direct possible pieces of evidence that thyroid cancer in children in these areas is related to exposure to isotopes released at the time of Chernobyl, and that these isotopes did not persist in the environment.

Radiation Studies

A number of measurements have been made to estimate the radiation dose received by the thyroid in children and adults in the exposed population. There are many difficulties in making a really accurate retrospective assessment of dosimetry. It may be more useful to relate the incidence of thyroid carcinoma to the known pattern of contamination and the known time taken for the radioactivity to reach that region, rather than making large-scale studies involving a number of assumptions in an attempt at reconstruction of the dosimetry of individuals. As mentioned above epidemiological studies could relate tumour incidence to factors that are likely to influence the thyroid dose. Research on biological measures of radiation exposure should be encouraged, in the hope of obtaining an objective assessment of the likely exposure in individual cases.

It is difficult to stress too strongly the importance of making a start as soon as possible on these and other research studies, and in particular in ensuring as soon as possible that the resected tissue from children with thyroid cancer presumed to be due to exposure to radioactive contamination from Chernobyl is handled and preserved in such a way that future research studies can be carried out. It is already likely to be impossible to carry out molecular biological studies on thyroid cancer due to exposure to Chernobyl occurring in children of 5 or 6 years of age. Next year it will be impossible to carry out studies on children of 7 or younger. The changes in these very young children may differ from those in older children and adults. Steps must be taken urgently to ensure that material is preserved.

## 11.C.	Coordination of the various Chernobyl related studies

A number of studies of the health effects of the Chernobyl accident are already underway. Some are largely concerned with humanitarian aid and the provision of equipment, whereas others are more focusing on scientific objectives. Most of these studies are directed to particular areas of the CIS or are aimed at a particular aspect of the problem. The Commission of the European Communities is one of the major international bodies that is well placed to make a major contribution to a comprehensive programme and to take initiatives for improvement of the coordination of existing programmes. With respect to the work relating to thyroid cancer in children, it is important to bring all appropriate experts together in order to formulate optimal medical and scientific solutions for diagnosis and treatment.

12. Conclusions

The Consensus Opinion of the Panel Members and Observers documents the agreement reached that there is a true increase in childhood thyroid cancer in areas around Chernobyl and that exposure to radioactive isotopes of iodine from the Chernobyl accident is the most likely cause of this increase. The Chernobyl reactor accident was unprecedented in scale, the consequent occurrence of thyroid cancer affecting young children is a tragedy which touches the emotions of all who are involved.

It was therefore proposed that urgent action is required to deal with both the humanitarian and scientific aspects of the problem. The following sections set out the recommendations and conclusions reached by the Panel on the actions that are required in both areas.

Technical and Humanitarian Assistance

A comprehensive project is urgently needed to deliver a complete package of facilities and training which will enable the Belarussian Ministry of Health to provide the optimal treatment for the childhood thyroid cancer patients. This package must include up-to-date equipment for the diagnosis, surgical treatment, and nuclear medical follow-up of the cancer patients as well as a continuing supply of all the necessary pharmaceutical and medicines to ensure a complete recovery and after-care.

Most of the surgical procedures are performed in the major referral centre in Minsk, where experienced surgeons are available, although operating theatres and other surgical facilities and equipment are not adequate. It is important to note that childhood thyroid cancer does not have to be a lethal disease if optimally treated.

The project must also include the training of medical specialists in Western hospitals and institutes in modern surgical techniques and in the use of modern diagnostic and therapeutic instrumentation which should be provided by the project. In addition the training programme should also allow for exchange visits of scientists and medical specialists in order to facilitate the introduction of the newer methods in the medical centres in Belarus.

The reported increase in childhood thyroid cancer in regions of the Ukraine suggests that a comparable Technical and Humanitarian Assistance Programme for the Ukraine will also be needed.

The Commission's "Technical Assistance to the Commonwealth of Independent States" (TACIS) Programme could be the ideal vehicle to achieve this desperately needed assistance, and the Radiation Protection Research Action, in collaboration with its contractors, is fully prepared to provide any specialised help which may be needed.

Research Cooperation

The occurrence of childhood thyroid cancer in the regions around Chernobyl is a tragedy but it offers an unique opportunity to study the molecular, cellular and biological characteristics and learn about the development of this radiation induced thyroid cancer. The importance of this information for radiation protection science cannot be underestimated. It is imperative that we learn all the lessons we can from the consequences of the accident so that we are optimally prepared for the future.

Childhood thyroid cancer is a rare disease and, although the treatment is well developed in the West, international guidelines for the treatment have not been defined. The optimisation of treatment protocols for surgery, follow-up and after-care of the young victims of this accident is of paramount importance.

The research cooperation must be based on an equal participation and a structured collaborative effort between scientists in the European Community and Belarus, the Ukraine and the Russian Federation.

The Radiation Protection Research Action collaboration with the CIS countries within the frame of the "Activités complémentaires de préparation, d'accompagnement et de suivi - Collaboration with the former Soviet Union in Radiation Protection" (APAS-COSU) programme offers the best possibility to achieve this research cooperative venture.

The implementation of both aspects of this proposal for assistance to Belarus and the Ukraine and the commitment of the scientific staff of the Radiation Protection Research Action, together with its contractors, will guarantee optimum interaction between the different facets of the humanitarian and scientific assistance programme.

References

Abelin, T., Averkin, J.I., Egloff, B., Furmantchuk, A.W., Gurtner, F., Kortkevich, J.A., Marx, A., Matveyenko, I.I., Okeanov, A.E., Ruchti, C., Schäppi, W. Childhood thyroid cancer in Belarus after the Chernobyl nuclear accident. To be published 1993.

Annals of the ICRP 1991.

Arntsing, R., Bjurman, B., De Geer, L., Edvarson, K., Finck, R., Jakobsson, S. and Vintersved, I. Field Gamma Ray Spectrometry and Soil Sample Measurements in Sweden Following the Chernobyl Accident, A Data Report. FOA Report D 20177-4.3. National Defence Research Establishment, Sundbyberg, Sweden, 1991.

Bartalena, L., Martino, E., Pacchiarotti, A., Grasso, L., Aghini-Lombardi, F., Buratti, L., Bambini, G., Breccia, M., Pinchera, A. Factors affecting suppression of endogenous thyrotropin secretion by thyroxine treatment analysis in athyreotic and goitrous patients J. Clin Endocrinol Metab, 64, 849-55, 1987.

Baverstock K.F., International Journal of Radiation Biology 50, iii-xii, 1986.

Belfiore, A., La Rosa, G.L., Padova, G., Sava, L., Ippolito, O., Vigneri, R. The frequency of cold thyroid nodules and thyroid malignancies in patients from an iodine-deficient area. Cancer, 60,3096-3102, 1987.

Briançon, C., Halpern, S., Jeusset, J., Fragu, P. Effects of various iodine intake on iodine thyroid autoregulation. Study with analytical ion microscopy and Iodine-129. Biol. Trace Element Res., 32; 267-273, 1992.

Ceccarelli, C., Pacini, F., Lippi, F., Elisei, R., Arganini, M., Miccoli, P., Pinchera A. Thyroid cancer in children and adolescents. Surgery, 104, 1143-48, 1988.

Dobbyns, B.M. and Hyrmer, A.B. The surgical management of benign and malignant thyroid neoplasms in Marshall Islanders exposed to hydrogen bomb fallout. World J. Surg, 16, 126-140, 1992.

Duffy, B.J. and Fitzgerald, P. Thyroid cancer in childhood and adolescence. J. Clin Endocrinol Metab. 1950, 10; 1296-1308.

Environmental transfer of radionuclides: implications of Chernobyl on terrestrial and aquatic ecosystems. Reports from a CEC Radiation Protection Research Programme Contractors Meeting held in Brussels on 25-26.6.1986 (unpublished results).

Evans, J.S., Moeller, D.W., and Cooper, D.W. Health effect model for Nuclear Power Plant Accident Consequence Analysis, Washington, Supt. of Documents; Springfield, Nat.Tech. Information Service. NUREG/CR-4124, S and 85-7185, 1985.

Franssilla, K.O., Harach, H.R. Occult papillary carcinoma of the thyroid in children and young adults. Cancer 1986, 58; 715-719.

Furmanchuk, A.W., Averkin, J.I., Egloff, B., Ruchti, C. et al. Pathomorphological findings in thyroid cancers of children from the Republic of Belarus. Histopathology 1992, 21, 401-408.

Gudiksen, P.H., Harvey T.F. and Lange, R. Chernobyl Source Term Estimation. In Proceedings of Seminar on Comparative Assessment of the Environmental Impact of Radionuclides Released during Three Major Nuclear Accidents: Kyshtym, Windscale, Chernobyl. EUR 13574. CEC, Luxembourg, 1991.

Hedinger, Ch., Williams, E.D. and Sobin, L.H. Histological typing of endocrine tumours. World Health Organisation, Geneva, 1988.

Hempelmann ,L., Hall, W.J., Phillips, M. et al. Neoplasms in persons treated with X rays in infancy. J. Natl Cancer Inst. 1975, 55; 519.

Holm, L.E., Dahlquist, I., Israelsson, A. and Lundell, G. Malignant thyroid tumours after iodine 131 therapy, a retrospective cohort study. New Engl. J. Med.1980, 303, 188-191.

Holm, L.E., Wiklund, K., Lundell, G. et al. Thyroid cancer after diagnostic doses of Iodine 131. J. Natl Cancer Inst. 1988, 80, 1132-1138.

International Commission for Radiological Protection, Publication No.60, 1991.

Johnson J.R. in "Age related factors in radionuclide metabolism and dosimetry" Eds G.B. Gerber, H. Metivier and Smith, H. Martinus Nijhoff Publishers, 249-260, 1987.

Lee, W., Chiacchierini, R.P., Shleien, B. and Telles, N.C. Thyroid tumours following ^{131}I or localised X irradiation to the thyroid and pituitary glands in rats. Radiation Research 1982, 92, 307-319.

Lindsay, S., Sheline, G.E., Potter, G.D., and Chaikoff, I.L. Induction of neoplasms in the thyroid gland of the rat by X irradiation. Cancer Research, 21, 9-16, 1961.

Lindsay, S., Nichols, C.W., Chaikoff, I.L., Induction of benign and malignant thyroid neoplasm in the rat. Arch Pathol. 81, 308-313, 1966.

Malone, J., Unges, J., Delange, F., Lagasse, R. and Dumont, J.E. Thyroid consequences of Chernobyl accident in the countries of the European Community. J. Endocrinol. Invest. 1991, 14, 701-707.

McWhirter, W.R., Petroeschevsky, A.L. Childhood Cancer Incidence in Queensland, 1979-88. Int J Cancer, 1990; 45: 1002-5.

Muir, C., Waterhouse, J., Mack, T., Powell, J., Whelan, S. Cancer Incidence in Five Continents. Vol. V. IARC Scientific Publications No.88. Lyon: International Agency for Research on Cancer, 1987.

Nagataki, S., Ingbar, S.H. Autoregulation: effects of iodine. In Braverman, L.E. and Utiger R.D. (eds.) Werner and Ingbar's: the Thyroid. Philadelphia, Lippincott Company, 306-312, 1991.

NCRP Report N° 80. Induction of thyroid cancer by ionising radiation. NCRP, 1985.

Pacini, F., Pinchera, A., Giani, C., Grasso, L., Baschieri, L. Serum thyroglobulin concentrations and 131-I whole body scans in the diagnosis of metastates from differentiated thyroid carcinoma (after thyroidectomy). Clin Endocrinol, 13,107-10, 1980.

Ramalingaswami, W., Iodine and thyroid cancer in man. In: Hedinger CE, ed. Thyroid Cancer. UICC Monograph Series, vol 12, Berlin: Springer-Verlag, 1969:111.

Report EUR 13199 Radiation Protection Research: Radiation Protection Programme Revision 1988-89; Post-Chernobyl actions, Executive summaries, 1990.

Report EUR 12551 Radiation protection Research: Feasibility of studies on health effects in western Europe due to the reactor accident at Chernobyl and Recommendations for research, 1990.

Ron, E., Modava, B., Preston, E. et al. Thyroid neoplasia following low dose radiation in childhood. Radiation Research 1989, 120; 516-531.

Ron, E., Lubin, J. and Schneider, A.B. Thyroid cancer incidence. Nature 1992, 360; 113.

Schlumberger, M., de Vathaire, F., Travaglia, J.P., et al. Differentiated thyroid carcinoma in childhood. J. Clin Endocr. Metab 1987, 65, 1088-1094.

Schneider, A.B., Shore-Freedman, E., Ryo, U. et al. Radiation induced tumours of the head and neck following childhood irradiation. Medicine 1985, 64; 1-15.

Shimaoka, K., Getag, E.P. and, Rao, U. Anaplastic carcinoma of the thyroid. New York State J. Med 1979, 79, 874.

Shore, R.E. Issues and epidemiological evidence regarding radiation induced thyroid cancer. Radiation Research 1992, 131, 98-111.

Stoutjesdijk, J.F. and Zoeteman, B.C.J., (1987) Radioactive Contamination in the Netherlands as a Result of the Nuclear Accident at Chernobyl. Report of the Coordinating Committee for the Monitoring of Radioactive and Xenobiotic Substances (CCRX) VROM 70431/6-87. Published by the Ministry of Housing, Physical Planning and Environment. The Hague. The Netherlands.

Taurog, A. Hormone synthesis: thyroid iodine metabolism. In Braverman, L.E. and Utiger R.D. (eds.) Werner and Ingbar's: the Thyroid. Philadelphia, Lippincott Company, 51-97, 1991.

The International Chernobyl Project - Technical Report, Assessment of Radiological Consequences and Evaluation of Protective Measures. Published by the International Atomic Energy Agency. Vienna, 1991.

Tscholl-Ducommun, J. and Hedinger, Ch. Papillary thyroid carcinoma, morphology and prognosis. Virchows Arch [A] 396, 19-39, 1982.

Williams, E.D. Endocrine tumours of the thyroid. In Hormone Related Tumours. Nagasawa, H and Abe K, ed, Springer Verlag, Berlin, 1981.

Williams, E.D. Dietary iodide and thyroid cancer, In Thyroid disorders associated with iodine deficiency and excess. R. Hall, J. Kobberling, eds. Serono Symposium Publications, Raven Press, NY, 1985.

Wynford-Thomas, D., Stringer, B.M.J. and Williams, E.D. Dissociation of growth and function in the rat thyroid during prolonged goitrogen administration. Acta Endocrinol. 1982, 101, 210-216.

Acknowledgements

The Panel wishes to acknowledge the special help of His Excellency V.S. Kazakov, Minister of Health of Belarus which made the October mission to Minsk so productive. The Panel would also like to pay tribute to the unstinting cooperation received from Professors E.P. Demidchik; L.N. Astakhova; E. Cherstvoy; Drs. A.W. Furmanchuk; J.I. Averkin, Mrs. N. Ievleva, and all their collaborators, as well as the many Ukranian and Russian scientists attending the Minsk Symposium.

Thanks are due to Drs. L.R. Anspaugh, G.W. Beebe, A. Bouville, J. Dumont, P. Hubert, Y. Riaboukhine, C. Ruchti, M. Schlumberger, G. Wagemaker, for their cooperation and contributions to the report.

The Panel would also like to thank Ms. N. Azpiri-Lcjardi, S. Gee and J. Van De Gaer for their administrative support.

ANNEX.   GLOSSARY

Absolute risk

The excess risk due to an agent such as radiation calculated by subtracting the frequency in unexposed individuals from that in exposed individuals. It is based on the assumption that the increased use of the agent depends on the dose but is not related to the underlying natural risk.

Absorbed dose

The amount of energy from radiation absorbed by a unit mass of tissue or other medium. One gray (Gy) is the equivalent of one joule of energy absorbed per kilogram (in older units 1 rad is 100 ergs absorbed per gram).

Activity

The level of radioactivity present defined by the number of atomic disintegrations in a set time. Each disintegration releases energy in the form of radiation. One becquerel (Bq) is one disintegration per second. One curie (Ci) is 3.7×10^{10} disintegrations per second.

Autoimmunity

The condition resulting from the development in an individual of an immune reaction against a constituent of their own body.

Baseline rate

The incidence of disease such as a cancer in a population which has not been exposed to the agent studied.

Becquerel

The amount of a radioactive substance defined not by weight but by radioactivity in terms of frequency of the atomic disintegrations that give rise to the radiation. One becquerel equals one disintegration per second.

Carcinoma

A cancer (malignant tumour) originating in epithelial tissue, for example, skin, intestines, or thyroid.

Case-control study

An investigation of a cause of a disease made by comparing the frequency of exposure of a group of patients who have the condition to a possible cause with the frequency of exposure that of a control group individually matched as far as possible in terms of variables other than the suspected cause.

Cohort study

An investigation of the cause of a disease made by identifying a group of patients exposed to the possible causative agent and studying the appearance of the disease in this group over a follow-up period in comparison to its appearance in a similar but unexposed group.

Curie

The amount of a radioactive substance defined not by weight but by its radioactivity in terms of the frequency of the atomic disintegration that give rise to the radiation. One curie equals 3.7×10^{10} disintegrations per second.

Dose effect (dose-response) model

> The relationship between the dose of radiation or other potential agent causing a disease such as cancer with the frequency or severity of the disease caused. response) depends on dose.

Dose equivalent

> A quantity that expresses, for the purposes of radiation protection and control, an assumed equal biological effectiveness of a given absorbed dose on a common scale for all kinds of ionizing radiation. SI units is the Sievert.

Dose rate

> The quantity of dose absorbed per unit time.

Dose Rate Effectiveness Factor (DREF)

> A factor by which the effect caused by a specific dose of radiation changes at low as compared to high dose rates.

Etiology

> The cause or origins of disease.

Fallout

> Radioactive debris from a nuclear detonation or other source usually deposited from air-borne particulates.

Gamma radiation

Short wavelength electromagnetic radiation of nuclear origin, similar to X rays but usually of higher energy (100 keV to 9 MeV). Also known as gamma rays.

Goiter

Enlargement of part or all of the thyroid gland.

Graves' disease

A disease state in which the thyroid gland enlarges and may produce excessive amounts of thyroid hormone. Currently considered to represent an autoimmune disease in which abnormal antibodies are made which mimic the effect of thyroid stimulating hormone. Also known as Basedow's disease.

Gray (Gy)

A measure of the amount of energy absorbed by tissue or other substance exposed to radiation. One Gy is equal to 100 rads, and represents one joule of energy absorbed per kilogram.

Half-life, biologic

Time required for the body to eliminate half of an administered dose of any substance by regular processes of elimination; it is approximately the same for both stable and radioactive isotopes of a particular element.

Half-life, radioactive

Time required for a radioactive substance to lose 50% of its activity by decay.

Hyperthyroidism

Functional, metabolic state caused by excess amounts of thyroid hormones.

Hypothyroidism

Functional, metabolic state caused by the failure of the thyroid gland to produce adequate amounts of thyroid hormone.

Incidence

Or incidence rate; the rate of occurrence of a disease within a specified period of time, often expressed as number of cases per 100,000 individuals per year.

In utero

In the womb, i.e., before birth.

In vitro

(Literally, in glass), in culture or in the test-tube (as opposed to in vivo, in the living individual).

Ionizing radiation

Radiation sufficiently energetic to dislodge electrons from an atom. Ionizing radiation includes x and gamma radiation, electrons (beta radiation), alpha particles (helium nuclei), and heavier charge atomic nuclei. Neutrons ionize indirectly by colliding with atomic nuclei.

Isotopes

Elements may have several isotopes, these are nuclides with the same number of protons in their nuclei, and hence the same atomic number. They differ in the number of neutrons, and therefore in the mass number. The chemical properties of isotopes of a particular element are usually identical.

Life-span study (LSS)

A study of the occurrence of disease throughout the lives of a defined group of individuals. In the life-span study of the Japanese atomic-bomb survivors; the sample consists of 120,000 persons, of whom 82,000 were exposed to atomic bomb radiation, mostly at low doses.

Mortality (rate)

The rate at which people die from a disease, e.g., a specific type of cancer, often expressed as number of deaths per 100,000 per year.

Person-gray

Unit of population exposure obtained by summing individual dose-equivalent values for all people in the exposed population. Thus, the number of person-grays contributed by one person exposed to one Gy is equal to that contributed by 100,000 people each exposed to $10\,\mu$Gy.

Rad

A unit of absorbed dose. Replaced by the Gray (Gy) in modern units.

Radioactivity

The property of some isotopes (nuclides) of spontaneously emitting radiation, either as subatomic particles or as gamma radiation, or as X radiation after orbital electron capture. Radioactive nuclides may also undergo spontaneous fission.

Radioisotope

An element may occur in several forms or isotopes, one or more of which may be a radioisotope. This is a radioactive atomic species of an element with the same atomic number and usually identical chemical properties to the stable non-radioactive form.

Radionuclide

A radioactive type or species of atom characterised by the constitution of its nucleus.

Radiosensitivity

Relative susceptibility of cells, tissues, organs and organisms to the injurious action of radiation; radiosensitivity and its antonym, radioresistance, are used in a comparative rather than an absolute sense.

Relative biological effectiveness (RBE)

Biological potency of one radiation as compared with another to produce the same biological endpoint. It is numerically equal to the inverse of the ratio of absorbed doses of the two radiations required to produce equal biological effect. The reference radiation is often 200-Kv x rays.

Relative risk

An expression of excess risk relative to the underlying (base-line) risk; if the excess equals the baseline risk the relative risk is 2.

Sievert

The unit of absorbed radiation dose modified to take account of its biological effectiveness. It is equal to the dose in Gy multiplied by a quality factor and by other modifying factors, for example, a factor related to distribution. One sievert (Sv) equals 100 rem.

Standard mortality ratio (SMR)

The ratio of the disease or accident mortality rate in a certain specific population compared with that in a standard population. The ratio is based on 100 for the standard so that an SMR of 200 means that the test population has twice the mortality from that particular cause of death.

Threshold hypothesis

The assumption that no radiation injury occurs below a specified dose.

Thyroglobulin

The specific protein synthesized by the thyroid follicular cells.

Thyrotropin (TSH)

The hormone secreted by the anterior pituitary gland that regulates thyroid gland function.

Thyroxine (T4)

The main hormone secreted by the thyroid gland.

Triiodothyronine (T3)

The most active form of thyroid hormone.

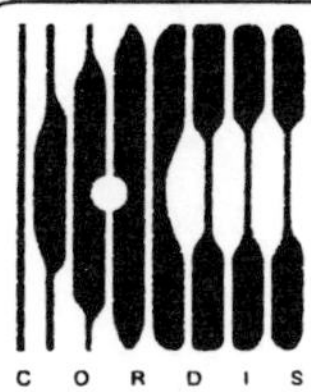

For up-to-date information on European Community research...

Community Research & Development Information Service

CORDIS is the Community information service set up under the VALUE programme to give quick and easy access to information on European Community research programmes. It consists of an on-line service at present offered free-of-charge by the European Commission Host Organisation (ECHO) and a series of off-line products such as:

- **CORDIS on CD-ROM;**
- **CORDIS Interface for *Windows* users;**
- **Multimedia Guide to *European Science and Technology*.**

The on-line databases can be assessed either through a *menu-based interface* that makes CORDIS simple to use even if you are not familiar with on-line information services, or for experienced users through the standard easy to learn *Common Command Language (CCL)* method of extracting data.

CORDIS comprises at present eight databases:

- RTD-News: short announcements of Calls for Proposals, publications and events in the R&D field
- RTD-Programmes: details of all EC programmes in R&D and related areas
- RTD-Projects: containing over 17,000 entries on individual activities within the programmes
- RTD-Publications: bibliographic details and summaries of more than 57,000 scientific and technical publications arising from EC activities
- RTD-Results: provides valuable leads and hot tips on prototypes ready for industrial exploitation and areas of research ripe for collaboration
- RTD-Comdocuments: details of Commission communications to the Council of Ministers and the European Parliament on research topics
- RTD-Acronyms: explains the thousands of acronyms and abbreviations current in the Community research area
- RTD-Partners: helps bring organisations and research centres together for collaboration on project proposals, exploitation of results, or marketing agreements.

For more information on CORDIS registration forms, contact:

CORDIS Customer Service
European Commission Host Organisation
BP 2373
L-1023 Luxembourg
Tel.: (+352) 34 98 12 40 Fax: (+352) 34 98 12 48

If you are already an ECHO user, please indicate your customer number.

European Communities — Commission

**EUR 15248 — Thyroid cancer in children living near Chernobyl
Expert panel report on the consequences of the
Chernobyl accident**

D. Williams, A. Pinchera, A. Karaoglou, K. H. Chadwick

Luxembourg: Office for Official Publications of the European Communities

1993 — VI, 108 pp., num. tab., fig. — 16.2 x 22.9 cm

Radiation protection series

ISBN 92-826-5515-6

Price (excluding VAT) in Luxembourg: ECU 13.50

In January 1992, under the Radiation protection research and training programme, a panel of experts was set up to evaluate the current situation
concerning reported increased rates of thyroid cancer in children living near
Chernobyl at the time of the nuclear reactor accident on 26 April 1986.

This report documents the findings of the panel with respect to the occurrence of childhood thyroid cancer in Belarus as of November 1992 and
makes strong recommendations for urgent technical and humanitarian
assistance and research cooperation.